Surgery at the Thoracic Outlet

General Editor, Wolfe Surgical Atlases:
William F. Walker, DSc, ChM, FRCS (Edin. and England), FRS (Edin.).

Single Surgical Procedures 23

A Colour Atlas of

Surgery at the Thoracic Outlet

Edgar W. Parry
MB, ChM, FRCS, FRCSE
Consultant General and Vascular Surgeon,
Broadgreen Hospital, Liverpool and
Lecturer in Clinical Surgery, University of Liverpool

Photography by Charles T. Fitz-Simon
Head of Medical Photography,
Eastern District Group of Hospitals, Liverpool

Wolfe Medical Publications Ltd

Published by Wolfe Medical Publications Ltd, 1985
Printed by Royal Smeets Offset b.v.,
Weert, Netherlands
ISBN 0 7234 1033 X

This book is one of the titles in the series of Wolfe Single Surgical Procedures, a series which will eventually cover some 200 titles.

If you wish to be kept informed of new additions to the series and receive details of our other titles, please write to Wolfe Medical Publications Ltd, Wolfe House, 3 Conway Street, London W1P 6HE.

We list below a few of the other titles in print and in preparation in the Single Surgical Procedures series. Titles already published are marked (⋆); those titles to be published during the coming months are marked (●).

⋆*Parotidectomy*
⋆*Traditional Meniscectomy*
⋆*Inguinal Hernias & Hydroceles in Infants and Children*
⋆*Surgery for Pancreatic & Associated Carcinomata*
⋆*Subtotal Thyroidectomy*
⋆*Anterior Resection of Rectum*
⋆*Boari Bladder-Flap Procedure*
⋆*Surgery for Varicose Veins*
⋆*Treatment of Carpal Tunnel Syndrome*
⋆*Seromyotomy for Chronic Duodenal Ulcer*
⋆*Surgery for Undescended Testes*
⋆*Operations on the Internal Carotid Artery*
⋆*Renal Transplant*
⋆*Lumbar Discography*
⋆*Visceral Artery Reconstruction*
⋆*Minor Operations on the Hand*
⋆*Flexor Tendon Repair*
⋆*Proctocolectomy*
⋆*Common Operations of the Foot*
⋆*Right Hemicolectomy*
⋆*Extra-cranial and Intra-cranial Anastomosis*
⋆*Surgery for Hirschsprung's Disease*
⋆*Thyroid Lobectomy*
●*External Fixation*
●*Anterior Cervical Spine Fusion*
●*Liver Transplantation*
●*Modified Radical Mastectomy*
●*Paratopic Transplant of Body and Tail of the Pancreas*
●*Subdiaphragmatic Total Gastrectomy for Malignant Disease*
●*Left Hemicolectomy*
Resection of Aortic Aneurysm
Ileo-Rectal Anastomosis
Techniques of Nerve Grafting and Repair
Surgery for Dupuytren's Contracture
Athrodesis of the Ankle
Surgery for Congenital Dislocation of the Hip
Femoral and Tibial Osteotomy
Maxillo-Facial Traumatology
Surgery for Chondromalacia Patellae
Stabilisation for Extensive Spinal Injury
Spondylolisthesis
Laminectomy
Gall Bladder Cholecystectomy
Repair of Prolapsed Rectum
Resection of Oesophagus
Splenectomy
Anterior Nephrectomy
Bladder Augmentation
Caecocystoplasty
Hiatus Hernia
Total Gastrectomy
Billroth 1 Gastrectomy
Billroth 2 Gastrectomy
Abdominal Incisions
Thoracotomy
Chronic Pancreatitis Operation
Surgery for Strictures in Common Bile Duct
Biliary Enteric Anastomosis
Partial Hepatectomy
Splenectomy
Right Hemicolectomy
Appendicectomy
Incisional Hernia
Lung Lobectomy
Lung Removal
Gastric Reconstruction
Surgery for Lymphoedema
Dialysis Techniques
Surgery for Thoracic Outlet
Haemorrhoids
Abdominoperineal Resection of Rectum
Rectosigmoid Resection
Non-resectional Surgery for Multiple Bowel Stenosis
Surgery for Anorectal Incontinence
Craniotomy
Parathyroidectomy
Arterial Injuries
Arterial Bypass Grafts in Leg
Visceral Vascular Occlusion
Varicose Veins Surgery under Local Anaesthesia
Aortofemoral Bypass
Aortoilac Disobliteration
Technique of Small Vessel Repair
Technique of Nerve Grafting and Repair
Microsurgery Techniques
Reimplantation of Ureters
Pyloric Stenosis in Children
Cleft Palate Surgery
Anorectal Malformation
Amputations of the Lower Limb
Anterolateral Decompression
Spinal Fusion
Scoliosis
Spinal Fusion for Low Back Pain
Recurrent Dislocation of Shoulder
Joint Replacement of Elbow
Joint Replacement of Wrist and Hand
Operative Fixation of Fractures of the Forearm
Joint Replacement at the Hip
Joint Replacement at the Knee
Arthrodesis of the Knee
Triple Arthrodesis
Amputations of the Upper Limb and Hand
Plastering Techniques
Operations for Peripheral Nerve
Compression Syndromes
Techniques of Tendon Transfer in the Upper Limb
Arthrodesis of the Wrist
Reconstructive Procedures of the Thumb
Minor Operative Procedures
Technique of Arthroscopy of the Knee
Management of Fresh Ligamentous Injuries of the Knee

Contents

Introduction

Surgery at the thoracic outlet is primarily concerned with relieving neurovascular compression at the space between the clavicle and the first rib.

If subclinical manifestations are included, there is an incidence of 35–40 per cent of compression in the community with a preponderence of women to men, in the ratio 3:1.

Rob and Standeven[1] in 1958 introduced the term 'thoracic outlet compression syndrome', describing a group of conditions often difficult to separate clinically. The syndrome includes:

Scalenus anterior syndrome
Cervical rib
Costoclavicular compression
Hyperabduction syndrome
Pectoralis minor syndrome
Fractured clavicle and callus formation
Subclavian vein thrombosis
Chronic intermittent subclavian vein compression
Neurological compression involving C8 T1 nerve roots

Thoracic outlet compression syndrome simplifies terminology but does not simplify diagnosis or management.

Clagett[2] in 1962 stressed the importance of the first rib in the syndrome, in that it formed the floor of the outlet, or acted as the lower blade of the scissors.

The clinical presentation can be entirely arterial, venous, neurological or any combination of the three. The compression may be simply caused by narrowing of the costoclavicular space, the subclavius muscle and tendon intervening, or may be complicated by the presence of other abnormalities, such as a cervical rib, fascial bands, anomalous muscles, anomalous first rib, or abnormalities of the clavicle after fractures or tumour formation.

Spasm of muscular structures or scarring of soft tissues after even minor injuries can exaggerate the compression and trigger off the often severe symptoms.

Compression of the subclavian artery presents two clinical groups:

Group 1. Simple intermittent arterial compression produced by exercise or position of the arm.

Group 2. Arterial compression complicated by arterial injury or disease in the form of:

(a) Atheroma
(b) Thrombosis
(c) Fusiform or saccular aneurysms

The main anatomical factors causing compression are:

(a) Cervical rib
(b) Scalenus anterior muscle
(c) Fascial bands
(d) Narrowing of the costoclavicular space.

The space is narrowed and the symptoms are aggravated by abduction and external rotation of the arm to 90 degrees (AER 90).

In Group 1, symptoms of ischaemic diffuse pain, numbness, fatigue, pallor and coolness are aggravated by abducting or raising the arm. Raynaud's syndrome in response to cold and exercise occurs and may be severe. It is doubtful if ulceration and gangrene occur in simple compression without intra-arterial disease.

Signs of arterial compression are absent when the arm is resting by the side in adduction. When the arm is abducted and externally rotated to 90 degrees (AER 90), the radial pulse is weak or absent and a bruit is heard below the outer third of the clavicle. The blood pressure falls as the arm is abducted and 20 mm Hg is a significant change.

In Group 2, the pathological changes of thrombosis, atheroma and aneurysm formation give rise to more severe and persistent symptoms, even to intractable pain and gangrene. The intra-arterial thrombosis associated with stenosis or dilatation is the source of distal emboli. It is important to remember that the clinical picture can be dramatic, with sudden marked ischaemia of the forearm and hand, or may be transient from microemboli lodging in digital arteries with small areas of focal necrosis.

The clinical signs are similar but more marked than in Group 1. In particular there is absent or lowered blood pressure and a persistent bruit in all positions of the arm. Whereas in Group 1, the clinical state may be tolerable, in Group 2 surgical treatment is imperative. Before any surgery is planned, aortic arch angiography is essential to ascertain the exact site of thrombus formation and to exclude disease in the brachiocephalic artery on the right side, and the first part of the subclavian artery on the left side.

Venous compression is less common and, although a number of anatomical structures have been implicated, the important site of compression is between the clavicle and the first rib with the subclavius muscle playing an important role. Compression can be present in adduction and abduction, although it is the latter position that usually produces or exaggerates the symptoms.

Subclavian vein thrombosis or 'effort thrombosis', in our experience, only occurs as a result of compression[3]. This is always demonstrable clinically and radiologically on the uninvolved side. This is a rare clinical condition and, although thrombectomy is occasionally successful treatment, it is unusual to find a suitable case.

It is fallacious to say that conservative management of subclavian vein thrombosis gives satisfactory results; 75 per cent of patients have residual symptoms and in 50 per cent the pain and oedema is so severe that any arm function is difficult. Many are compelled to change their occupation.

Chronic intermittent subclavian vein compression is a distinct clinical entity, giving rise to serious disability. It causes discomfort, pain, swelling and cyanosis of the hands and forearms, in response to exercise at work, leisure activities such as swimming and repetitive movements when playing a musical instrument such as the piano or the violin. The superficial venous pattern may be prominent and more obvious in abduction. The external jugular vein characteristically fills and distends in abduction and empties in adduction. Compression doubles or trebles the venous pressure in abduction. Flow records show obliteration of flow in abduction, corresponding to the high pressure readings. Venography demonstrates obstruction at the costoclavicular level with dilated distal veins. Collateral veins may be seen in abduction and sometimes in adduction. Doppler tests show reduced or absent flow in abduction followed by a rushing flow as the arm is lowered to the side.

Neurological problems are more difficult to diagnose with certainty, especially when the only symptom is intermittent pain. The pain is characteristically in the (C8–T1) ulnar nerve distribution. The pain is brought on by repetitive movements of the arms, particularly when abducted. Daily work of typing, polishing, driving the car, brushing the hair, etc, become difficult. More severe neurological damage interfering with motor conduction gives rise to selective muscle atrophy and weakness in the hand. The first muscle to be affected is the medial head of the adductor pollicis, then the muscles of the hypothenar eminence and the interossei muscles. This condition is progressive but can be halted by surgery, though not necessarily producing any dramatic improvement in muscle function. The causative lesion is usually a fascial band or cervical rib.

Autoimmune and collagen diseases account for severe Raynaud's syndrome in the hand, and although treatment is primarily directed at the underlying disease, the distal ischaemic pain can be helped by carrying out cervicodorsal sympathectomy.

Buerger's disease, a nicotine sensitive condition causing ischaemic distal lesions in the fingers, can be arrested and healing promoted by cervicodorsal sympathectomy once the tobacco habit is halted.

Finally the embarrassing problem of hyperhidrosis can be cured by cervicodorsal sympathectomy.

The surgical procedures described in detail are:
Cervicodorsal sympathectomy
Excision of a cervical rib
Excision or division of fascial bands
Principles of arterial procedures at the thoracic outlet
Excision of the first rib – anterior and transaxillary approaches.

Supraclavicular anatomical exposure

All the supraclavicular procedures depend on detailed, careful anatomical dissection and exposure before any definitive operation is carried out. Poor technical and rough surgery will pay the penalty of severe and sometimes intractable postoperative pain. Dense scarring is liable to occur, with pain and stiffness around the shoulder, and this can be minimised by restricting movements of the shoulder for one month. Immediately postoperatively, the arm is strapped to the side for three or four days, and thereafter it is placed in a sling or collar and cuff, allowing movements at the elbow, wrist and hand only for four weeks. Undue traction on the roots and trunks of the brachial plexus by retractors is the most important cause of postoperative paraesthesia and pain. The roots and trunks of the plexus must be isolated carefully by dividing connective tissue between them and the nerves can then be separated and held apart with slings without tension. During the procedure, careful vigilance is essential to avoid over-enthusiastic pulling or retraction by the assistant. Complete and careful haemostasis is mandatory for ease of identification of all structures, and also to prevent postoperative haematoma – another cause of dense, woody postoperative scarring. The exposure described is common to all the operative procedures mentioned apart from trans-axillary resection of the first rib.

1

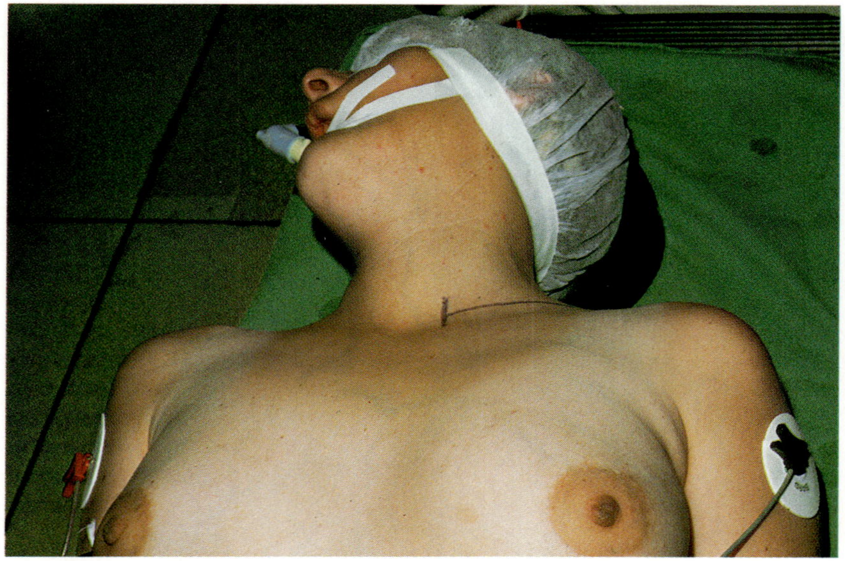

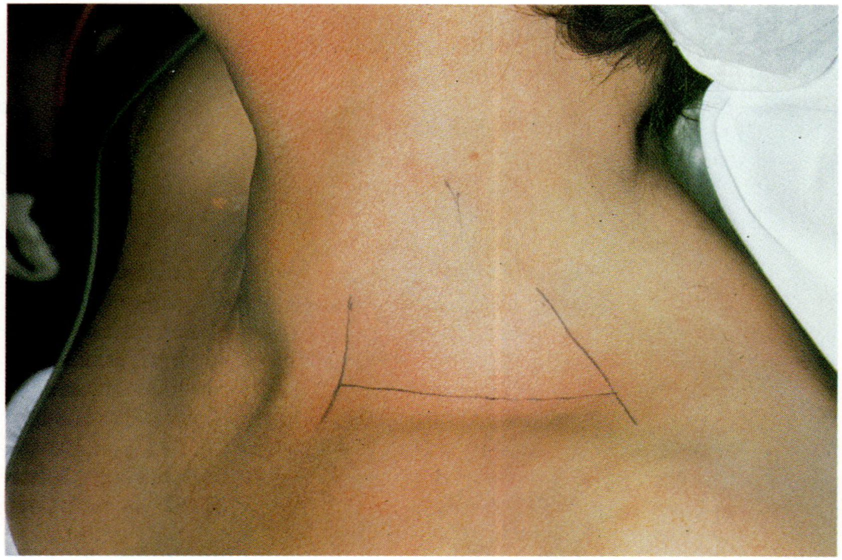

2

Exposure

1 Position of the patient on the operating table. The patient lies in a supine position, with a small sandbag placed longitudinally between the shoulders. The head is placed on a ring, or headrest, and turned to the opposite side. The arm on the operation side is pulled down and anchored to the side, thereby helping to open the supraclavicular fossa. A reversed Trendelenberg of 15 degrees is advised to avoid venous distension.

2 Marking the skin incision. The skin incision is marked 1 cm above and parallel with the clavicle. It extends from the sternal attachment of the sternomastoid muscle to the anterior border of the trapezius muscle.

3

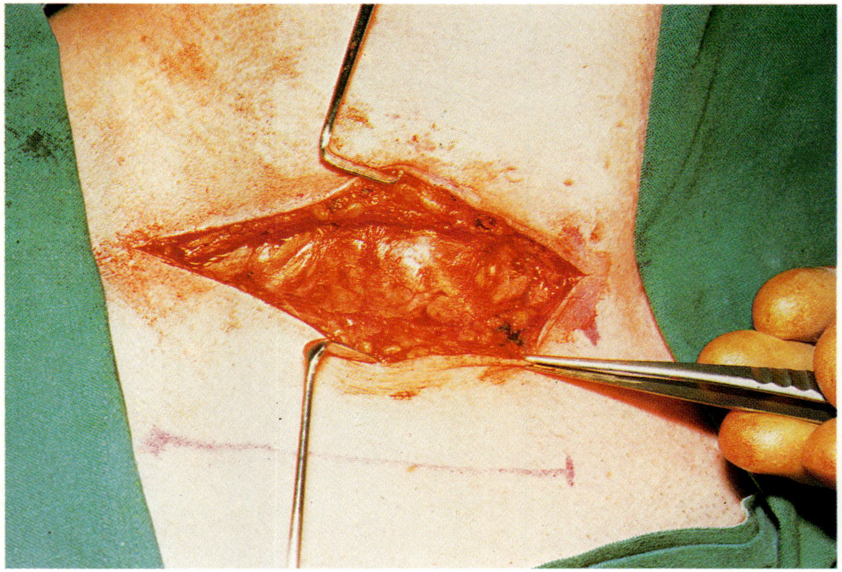

4

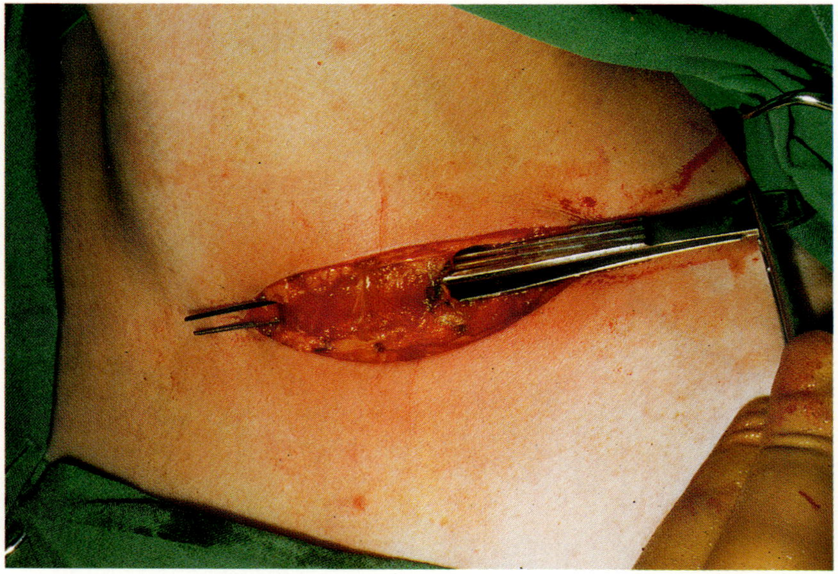

3 Incision of skin and platysma. The skin, superficial fascia and platysma muscle are incised. Infraclavicular nerves and small blood vessels are cut. Complete haemostasis is important before the next step.

5

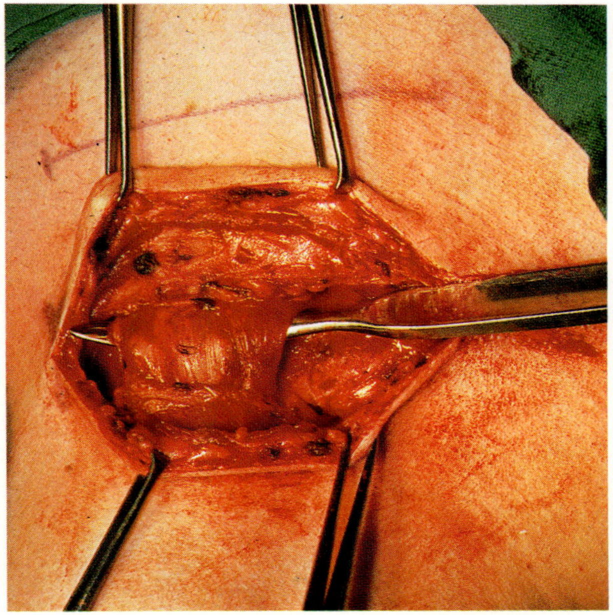

4 and 5 Division of deep fascia and sternomastoid muscle. The deep fascia is divided in the line of the incision and the posterior border of the broad clavicular head of the sternomastoid muscle cleared.

The anterior edge of the muscle, or the gap between the sternal and clavicular heads is defined. Scissors or blunt forceps can now be passed with ease behind the muscle while it is divided, and again absolute haemostasis obtained. A remnant of muscle is left on the lower end for resuturing at the end of the operation. The bulk of the muscle varies greatly from patient to patient, as seen in these two figures.

6 Defining the boundaries of the supraclavicular triangle. The internal jugular vein is now visible on the medial side of the field. A pad of fat (rarely described), varying in bulk from case to case, lies in front of the structures in the supraclavicular triangle. The posterior belly of the omohyoid muscle is seen passing obliquely downward from the medial to the lateral side, forming the upper boundary of the triangle.

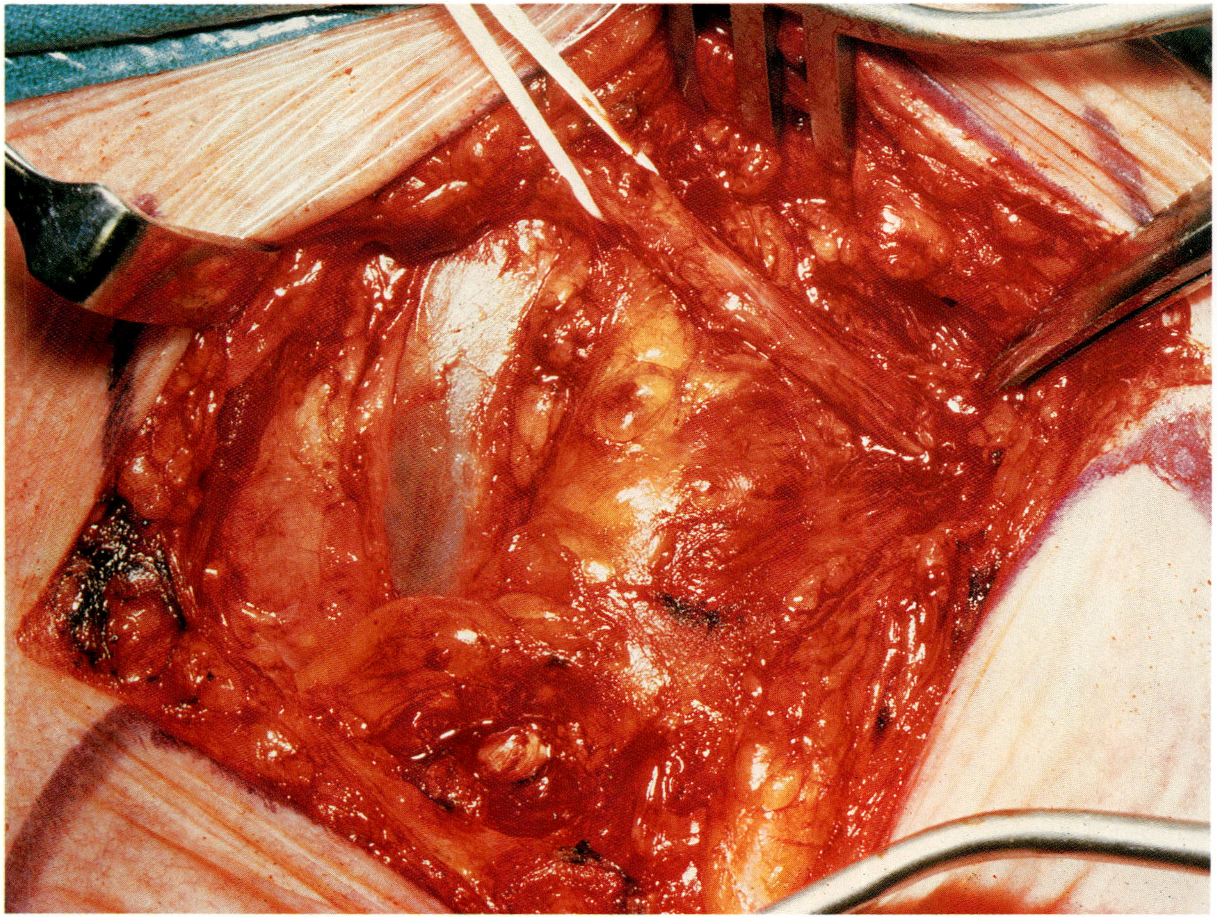
6

7 Dissecting the supraclavicular pad of fat. The pad of fat is dissected carefully from below upwards; **this step must not be hurried so as to maintain haemostasis by coagulation as dissection progresses, and to prevent damage to important underlying structures.** The dissection displays the lower part of the brachial plexus laterally, the external jugular vein passing medially, and in the lower medial corner the thoracic duct is seen at an earlier stage than usual.

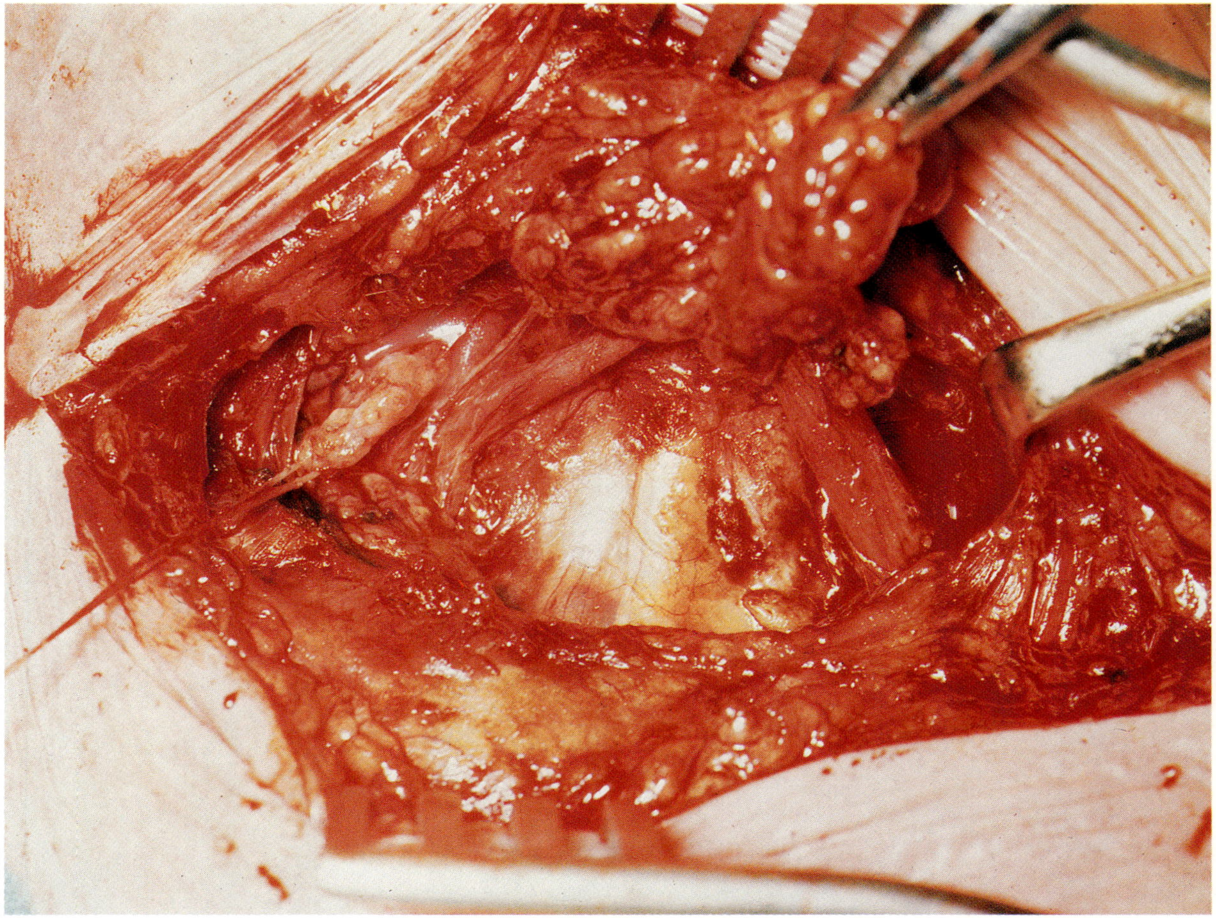

7

8 Displaying the contents of the supraclavicular triangle. Further dissection of the fat shows the brachial plexus clearly and the thick scalenous anterior muscle in the centre of the field. The suprascapular artery crosses the muscle from within outwards and can be ligated and divided at this stage. **The artery may not be seen at all during the operation as it may be at a lower level hidden behind the clavicle.**

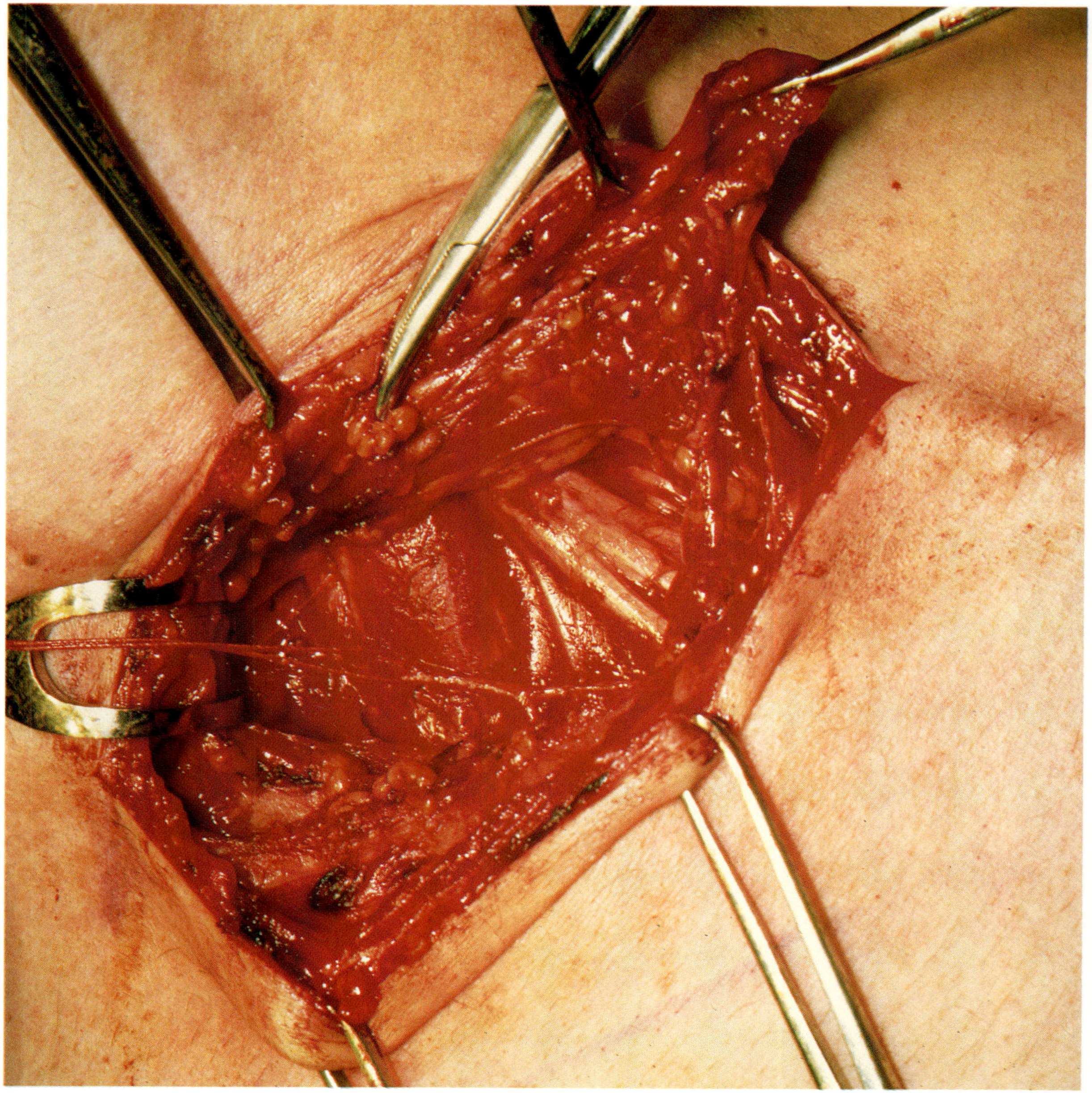

8

9 Dissection to free the transverse cervical artery and phrenic nerve. The transverse cervical artery is in the upper part of the triangle, buried in the pad of fat and lifted with it. **It is easily injured and can cause troublesome bleeding.** It must be dissected out of the fat, preserved or preferably formally ligated on the medial side and divided. Note the phrenic nerve lying within the fascia of the muscle and crossed by the transverse cervical artery. The pad of fat is retracted upwards and can be packed behind the omohyoid muscle. If visualisation of the anatomy is difficult, the omohyoid can be divided and further dissection of the fat carried out to improve the exposure.

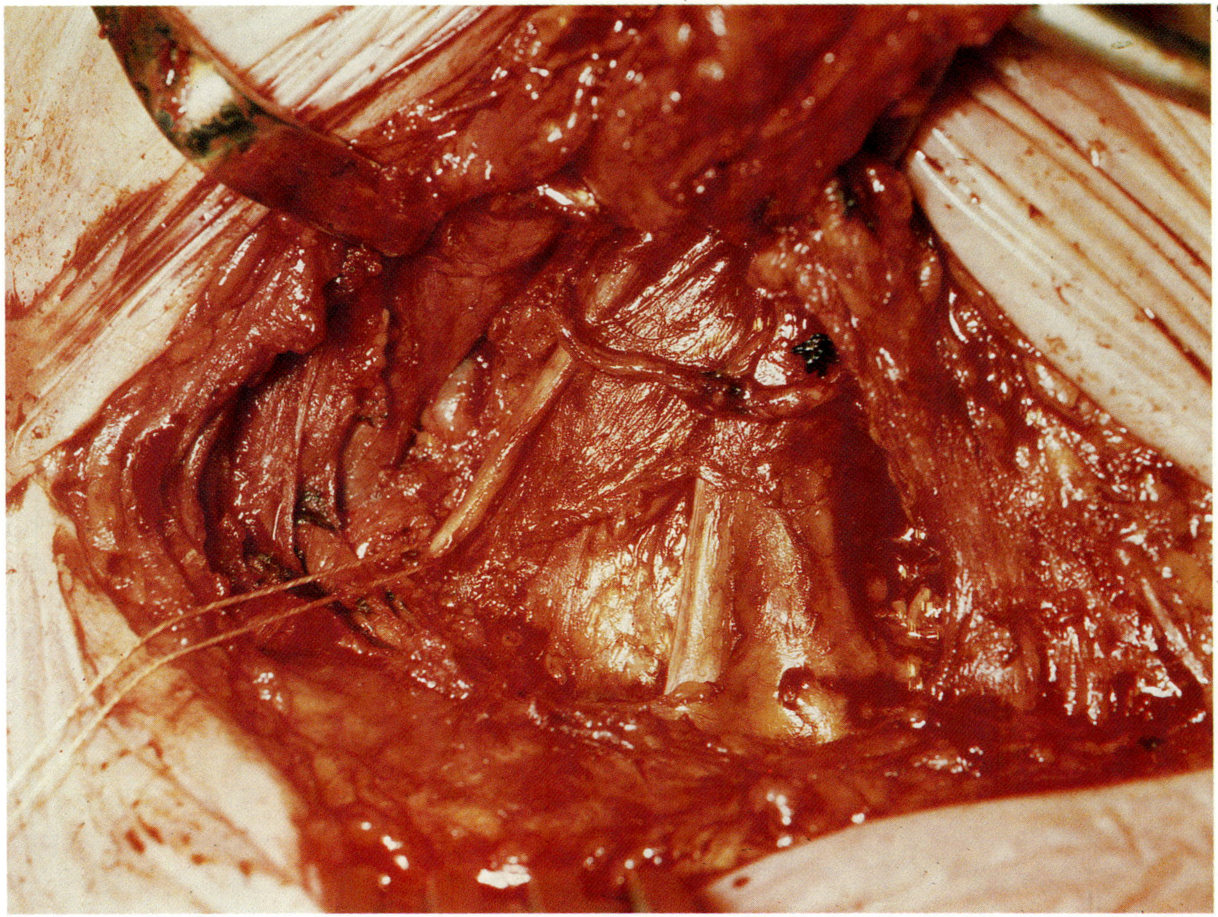
9

10 Orientation of the contents of the supraclavicular triangle. Orientation of the contents of the supraclavicular triangle is now imperative. The scalenus anterior muscle is the dominant structure. **No attempt is made to define its boundaries, or start any dissection to divide it, without first identifying the phrenic nerve lying within the fascia of the scalenus anterior.** It passes downwards and medially to disappear behind the subclavian artery and the internal jugular vein. If the nerve is not immediately visible, it will be found medially and slightly posterior to the medial edge of the muscle and possibly covered by muscle fibres.

The nerve is carefully lifted off the muscle and freed for the whole length of the field. This allows the nerve to be held aside gently and not forcibly retracted. Note the position of the nerve to the transverse cervical artery and internal jugular vein.

Dissection in the lower medial corner may damage the thoracic duct. This is seen easily if looked for and must not be damaged because of the dangers of producing a persistent lymph fistula.

On the lateral side of the triangle lie the roots and three trunks of the brachial plexus, covered at this stage by connective tissue. The subclavian artery is not usually visible at this stage, but its position is noted by palpation medial and lateral to the scalenus anterior.

In the presence of a cervical rib, the artery rises higher in the neck to arch over the rib as it curves downwards between the rib and the muscle.

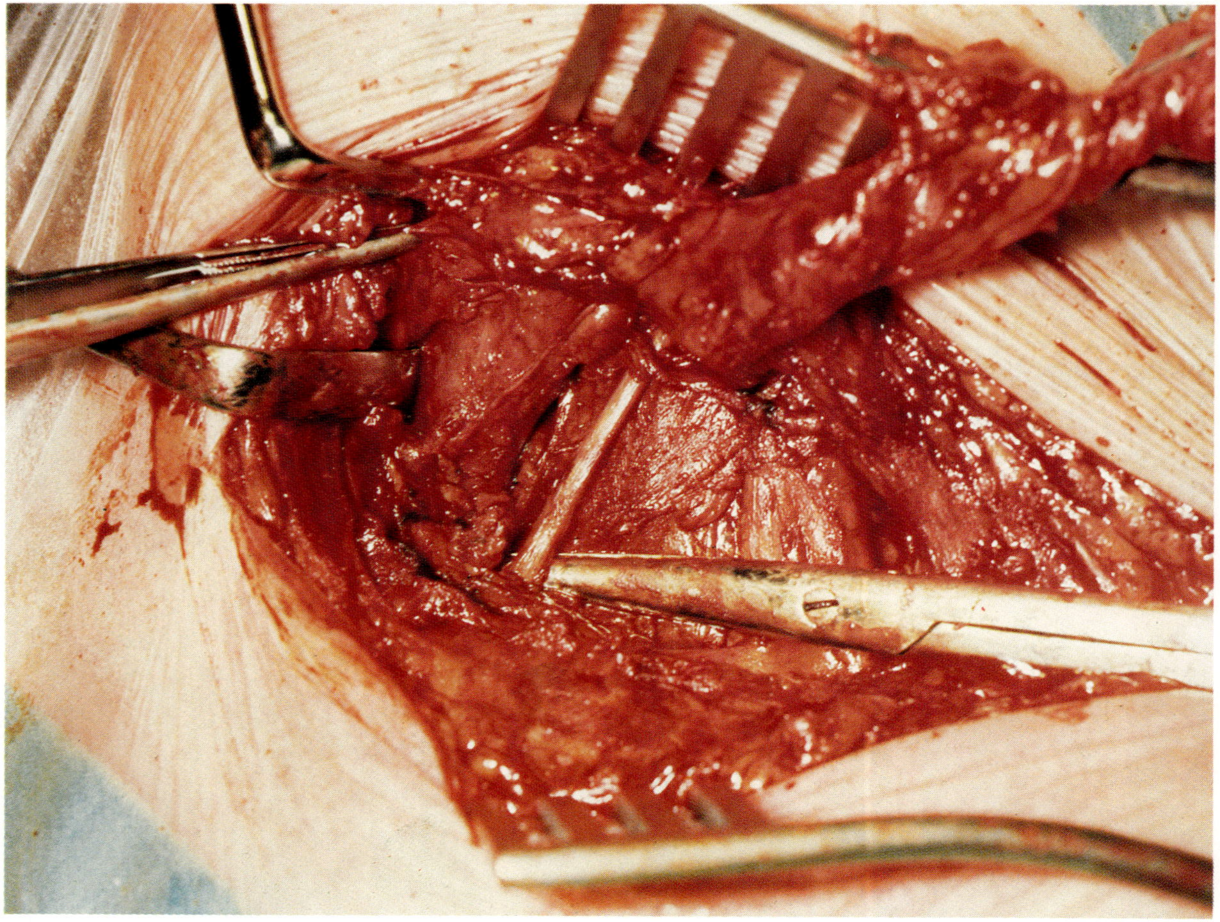
10

11 Identifying the position of the subclavian artery and defining the borders of the scalenus anterior muscle. In this figure, the artery has been identified lateral to the muscle and a soft sling passed around it. Knowing the position of the artery gives more confidence in clearing the muscle along its borders and posteriorly. A Lahey forceps is useful to pass gently behind the muscle to create a space through.

11

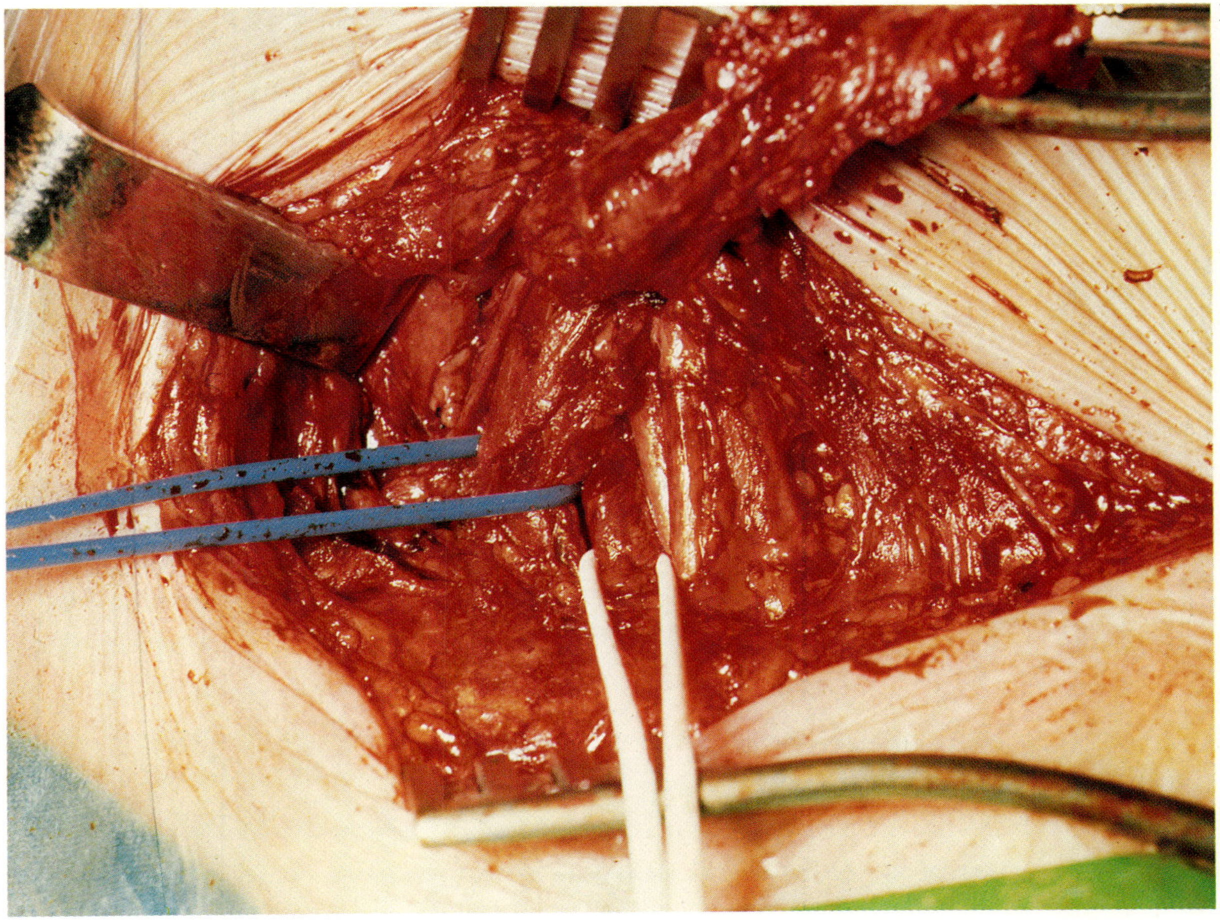

12

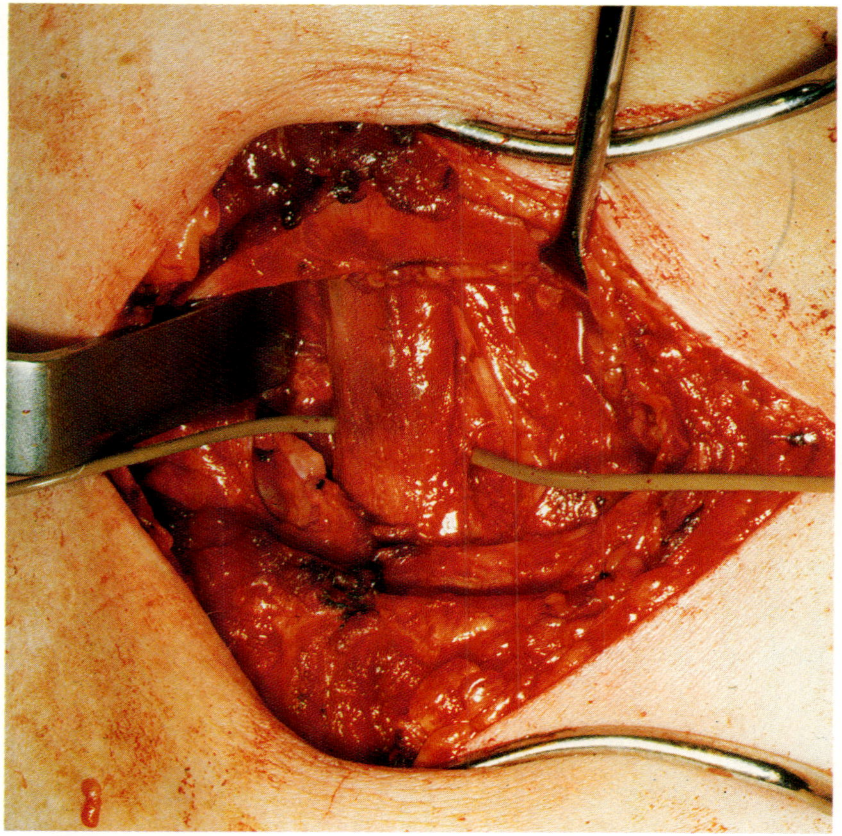

13

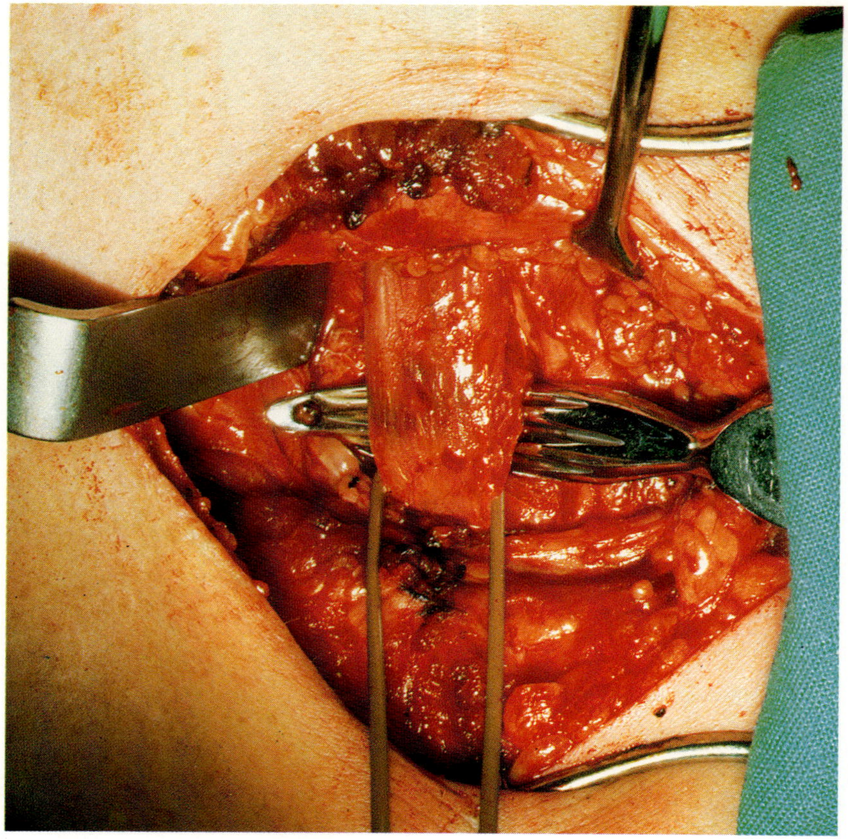

12 and 13 The borders of the scalenus anterior cleared and a sling passed behind, ensuring a safe layer for dividing the muscle. A blunt thyroid guide is passed behind the muscle. This important manoeuvre protects the artery before the muscle is divided close to its attachment to the first rib. The blood supply to the muscle is on its deeper aspect and can be anticipated and coagulated. **I always carry out total excision of the divided ends of the scalenus anterior from the field to avoid unnecessary scarring around the brachial plexus postoperatively.**

Dissection of the subclavian artery and its local branches (**14, 15** and **16**)

14 After division of the scalenus anterior muscle, attention is turned to the subclavian artery. The first step is to clear the artery laterally to pass a Lahey's forceps behind it and then put a soft plastic sling around it. This gives a measure of control. **I must stress that the subclavian artery is curiously thin-walled and friable compared with arteries of a similar size. It does not tolerate rough or careless handling. Horrendous haemorrhage from operative trauma has been recorded and no-one frequently operating in this area has not experienced worrying bleeding at some time or other.**

Dissection proceeds along the superior border of the artery to display the thyrocervical trunk, the smaller costocervical branch and other minor vessels. All these branches, regardless of small size, are divided between two fine thread ligatures 0.5 cm from the parent artery. **Artery forceps must not be used. This again gives a measure of safety because the branches are also friable and ligatures can cut through their walls. If this happens on or near the subclavian wall, brisk bleeding occurs, which is difficult to control. Cross-clamping of the artery may be necessary and formal repair suturing performed. Even this is fraught with dangers of further arterial wall damage. Precaution is all-important.**

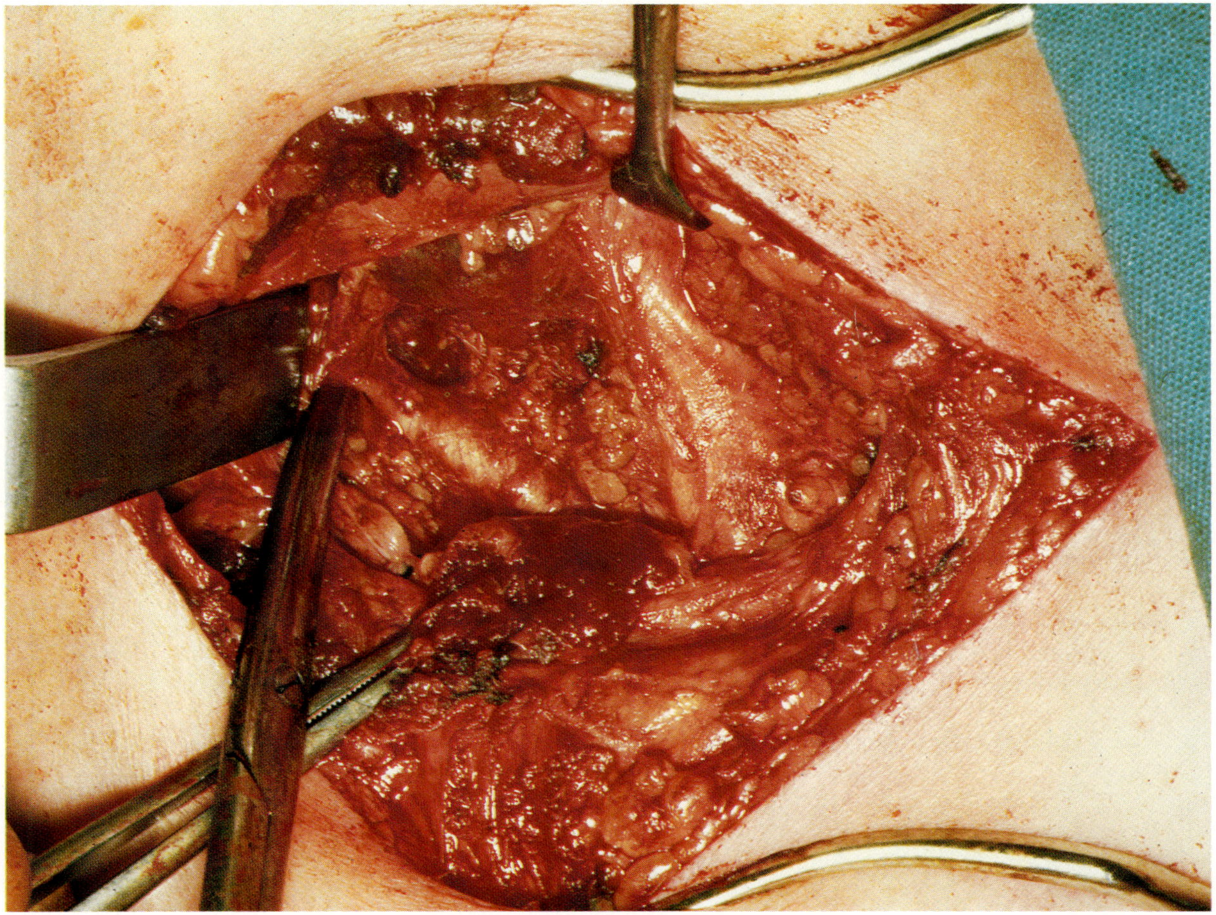

14

15

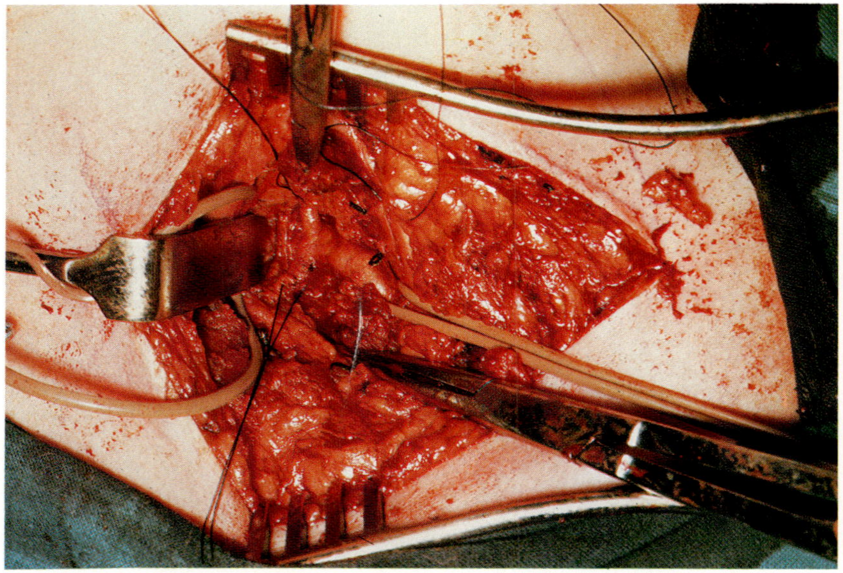

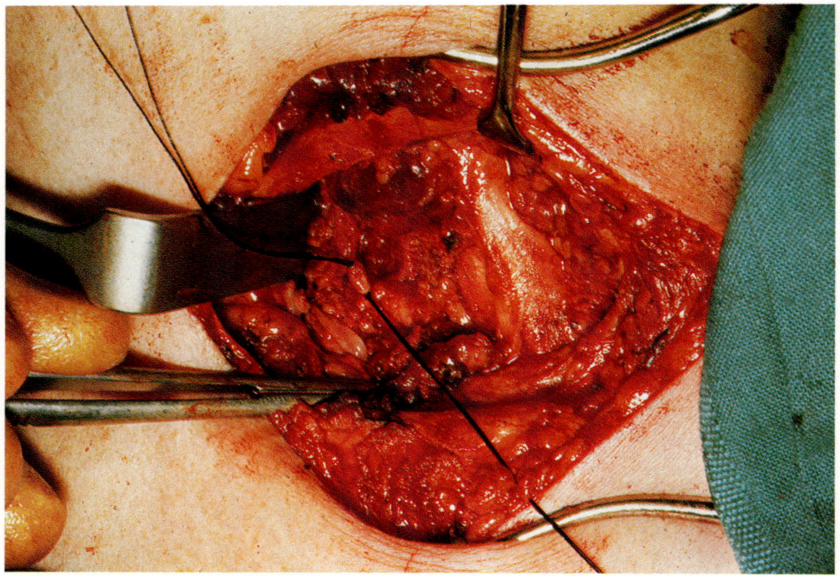

16

15 Shows ligatures around the thyrocervical trunk superiorly and the internal mammary artery inferiorly.

16 Two ligatures tied around the thyrocervical trunk and no artery forceps.

17 Retraction of subclavian artery downwards to reveal Sibson's fascia. After dividing the branches, the subclavian artery can be isolated from the surrounding connective tissue and displaced downwards without danger. At this stage Sibson's fascia, with the dome of the pleura behind it, can be visualised.

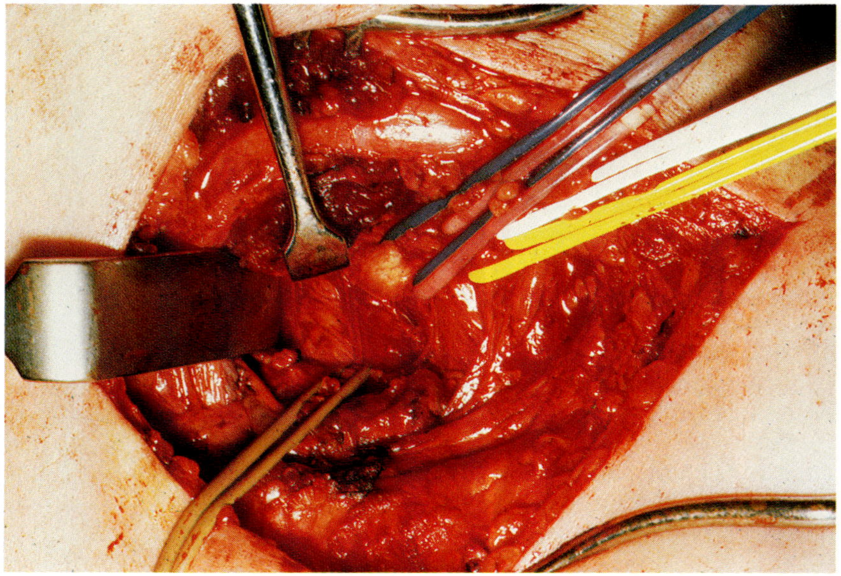

17

18 Dissection of the roots and trunks of the brachial plexus. The last anatomy to look at in the exposure phase is the brachial plexus. C5,6,7,8, and T1 roots can be identified. T1 root may present difficulty as it lies directly behind C8 root and can also be covered by muscle fibres lateral to the scalenus anterior. It is safe and simple to free the individual roots and the upper, middle, and lower trunks by dividing the connective tissue between them. Soft plastic slings are placed around the roots and trunks, allowing them to be held apart, rather than forcefully retracted with metal retractors. **I would recommend all young surgeons to familiarise themselves with this procedure, because there is no doubt that rough retraction and handling is the cause of postoperative pain and paraesthesia, which can be intractable and disabling. Similarly, lack of formal identification has led to injury of one or more nerve roots with severe disability and serious medicolegal consequences.**

The exposure described is common to all the definitive procedures at the thoracic outlet and make these infinitely easier and safer.

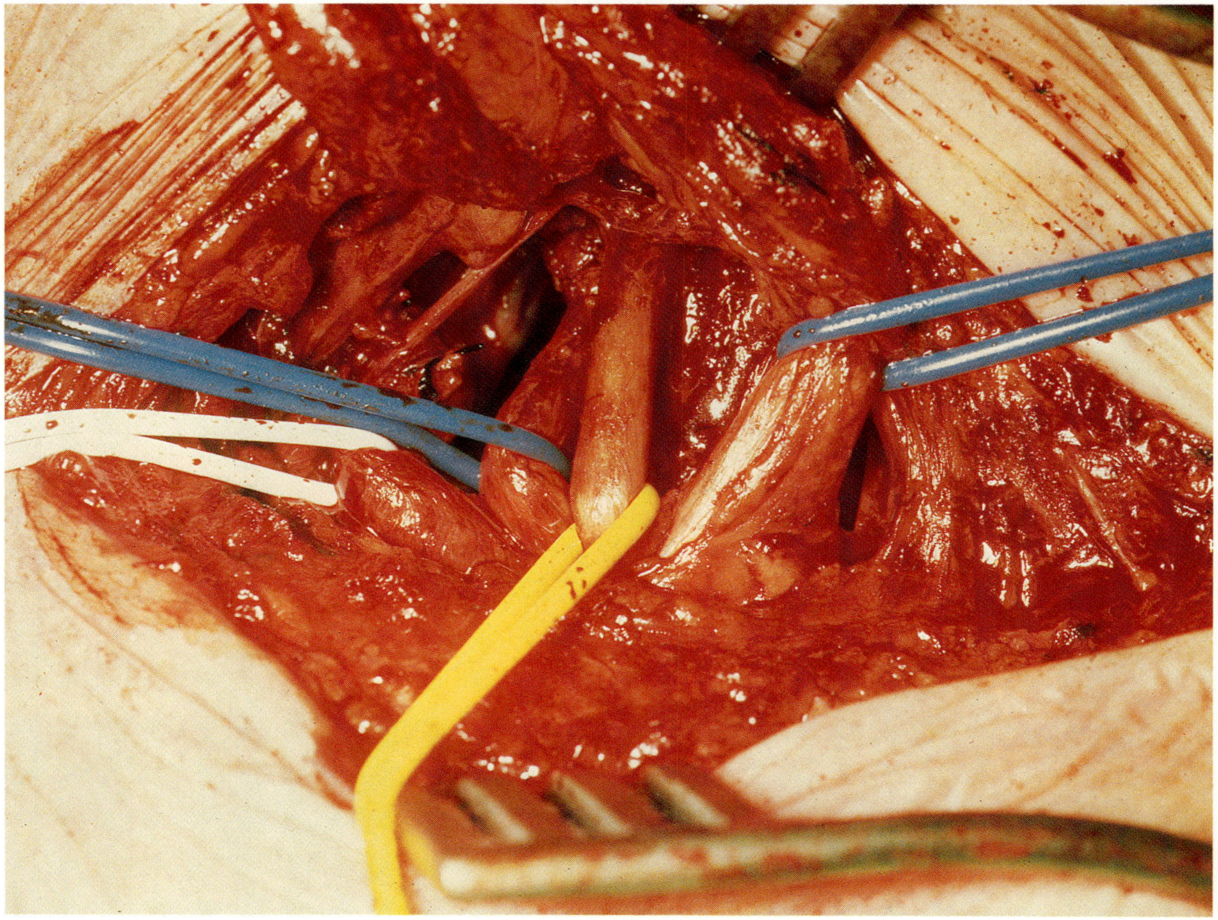
18

Cervicodorsal sympathectomy

Cervicodorsal sympathectomy is the commonest operation in this area to be carried out by a general surgeon. There is no complete agreement among surgeons as to the exact procedure or extent of the operation. The controversy centres around the stellate ganglion, a composite ganglion of the first thoracic and inferior cervical ganglia.

Total sympathetic denervation of the arm needs removal of the stellate ganglion but this results in a Horner's syndrome, because nerve fibres to the dilator pupillae and levator palpebrae muscles are removed. Excising the first thoracic ganglion or lower part of the stellate ganglion should not produce a Horner's syndrome, but it is often difficult to define the limits of this ganglion and to accidentally cause a Horner's syndrome. Fortunately many of them make partial or complete recovery in time. For most purposes the arm is sufficiently denervated by removing the second and third thoracic ganglia and sympathetic trunk together with the lower pole of the stellate ganglion. The indications for performing a cervicodorsal sympathectomy are:

1 As an adjunct to decompression of the thoracic outlet especially excision of a cervical rib where there is associated disease of the subclavian artery with distal embolic lesions and focal necrosis.
2 The relief of severe pain and ischaemia associated with advanced collagen or autoimmune diseases, especially scleroderma. Total stellate ganglionectomy with Horner's syndrome is sometimes acceptable in order to help these patients.
3 The management of Buerger's disease to promote healing of distal digital lesions after nicotine abstinence.
4 Hyperhidrosis.
5 Sudek's dystrophy and causalgia.
6 Raynaud's syndrome in the absence of background disease if the symptoms are frequent and distressing. Long-term abolition of symptoms, however, cannot be guaranteed.

19

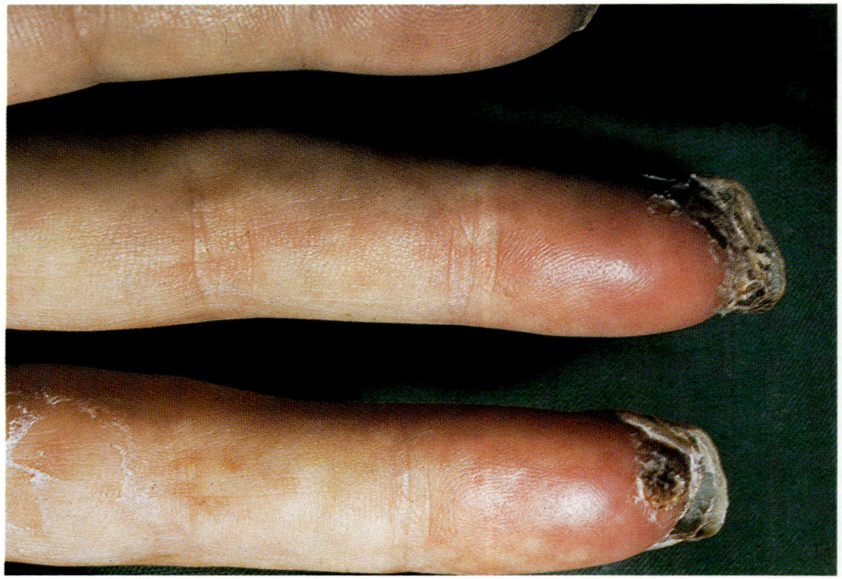

19 Distal focal necrosis caused by microemboli from thrombus in the subclavian artery.

20

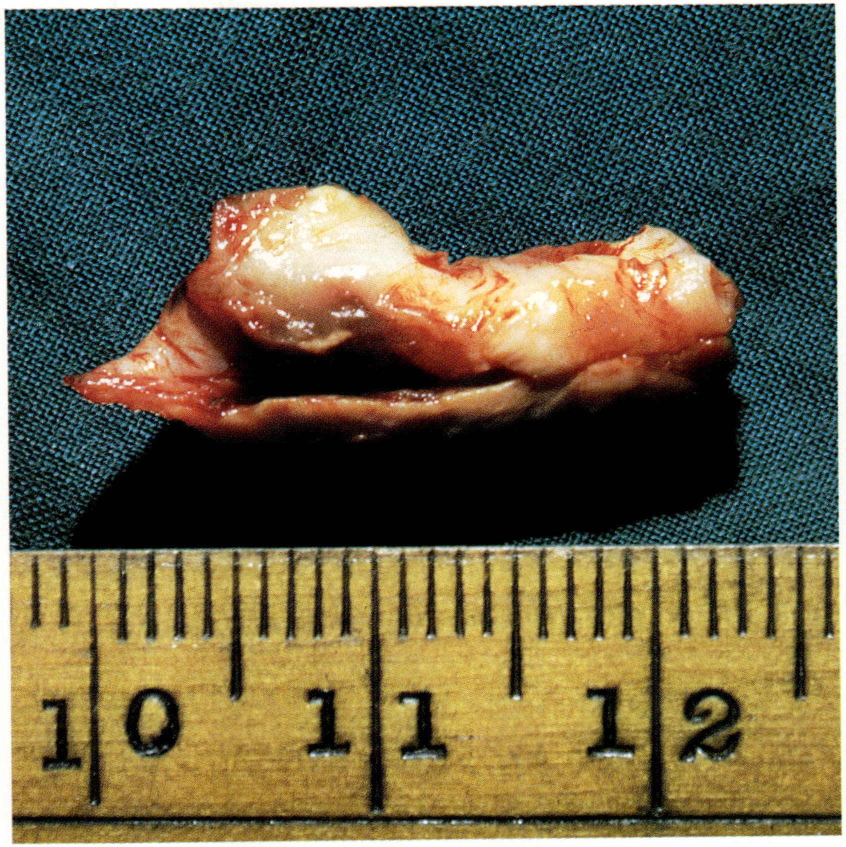

20 Thrombus within a resected fusiform aneurysm.

21

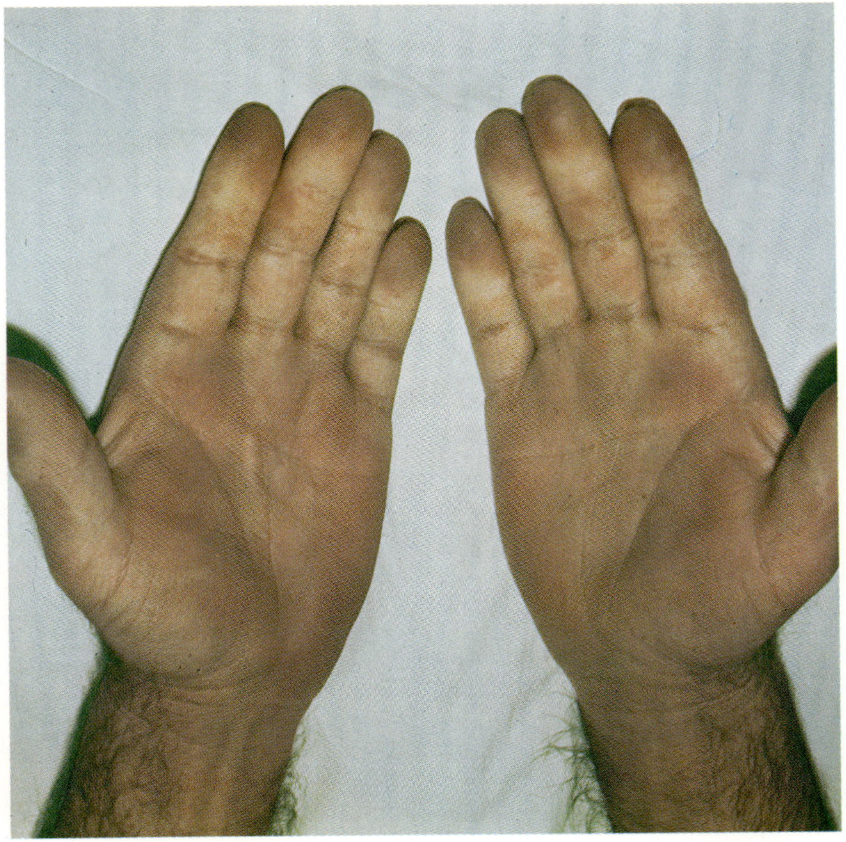

21 Pale ischaemic fingers with cyanosed terminal phallanges in scleroderma.

22

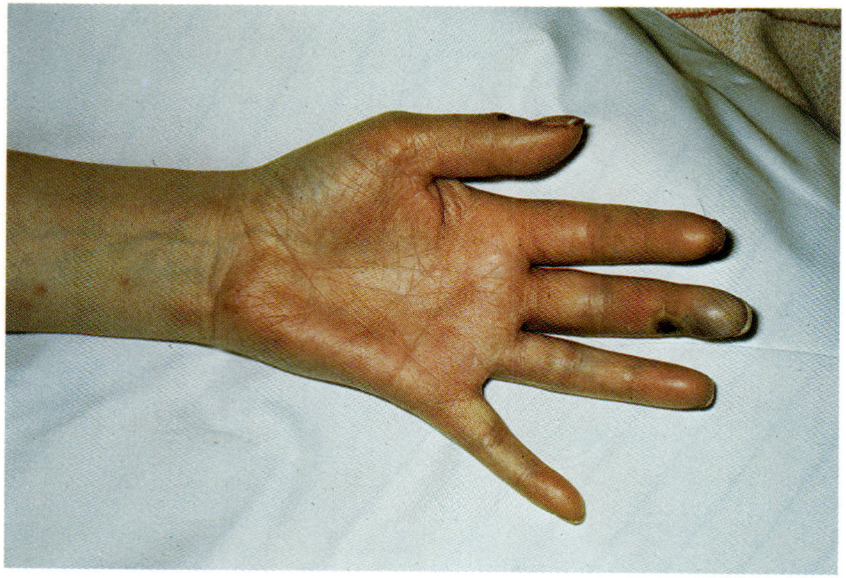

23

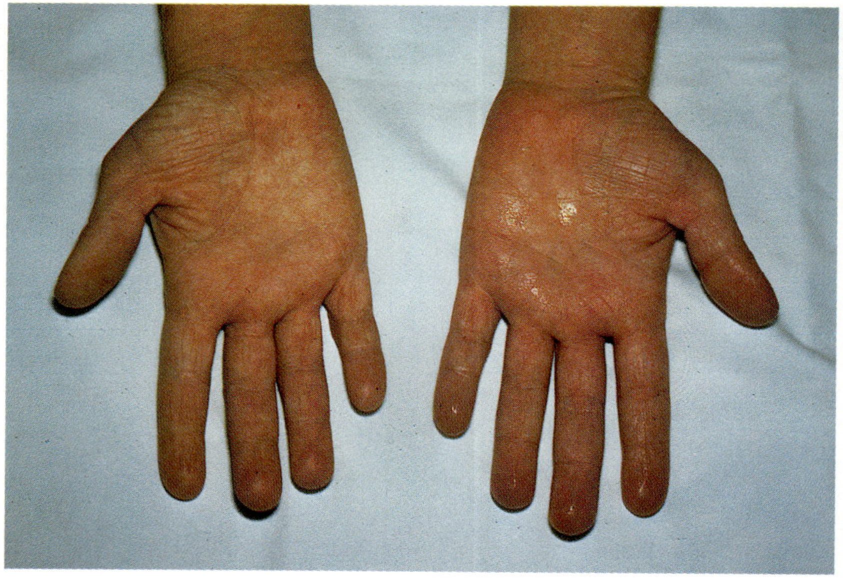

24

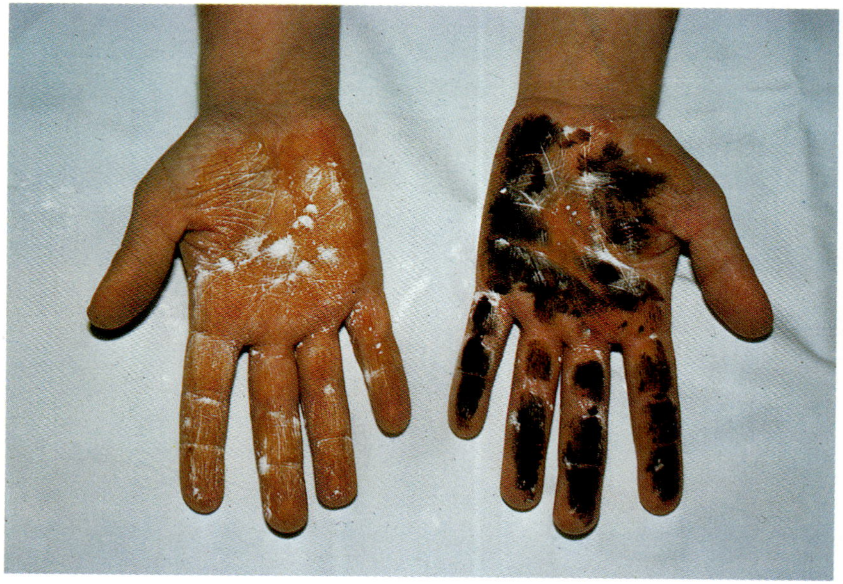

22 More advanced state of scleroderma with thin pointed fingers and local gangrene; note the tight, shiny, smooth skin of the fingers.

23 and 24 The next two illustrations show classical hyperhidrosis. The right hand has had cervicodorsal sympathectomy and is dry. The left hand shows marked sweating. The second illustration shows the positive starch-iodine test in the left hand.

25

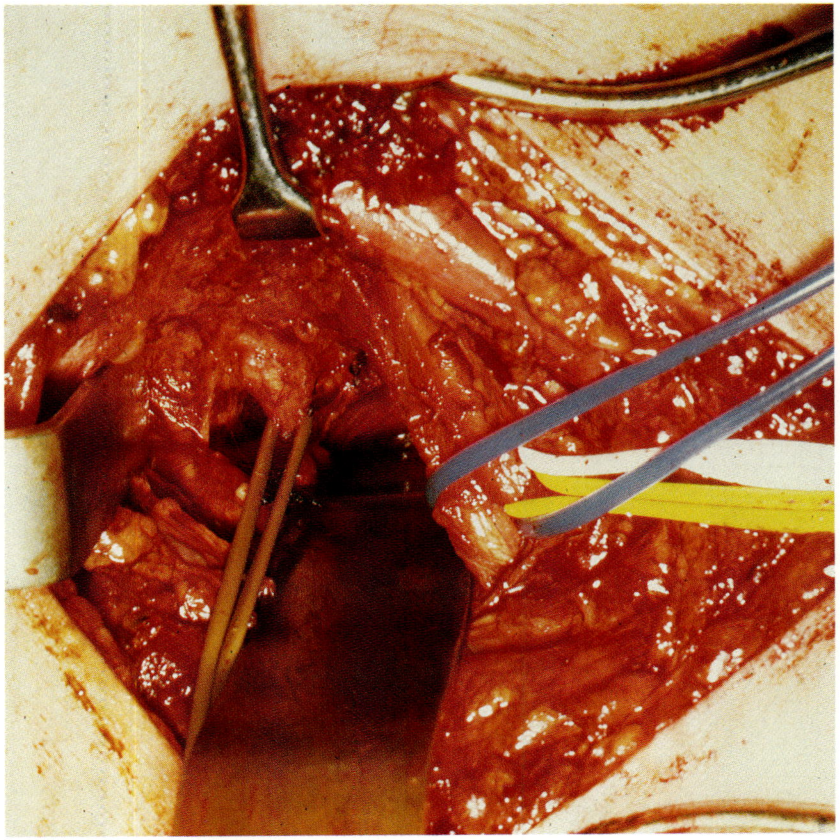

26

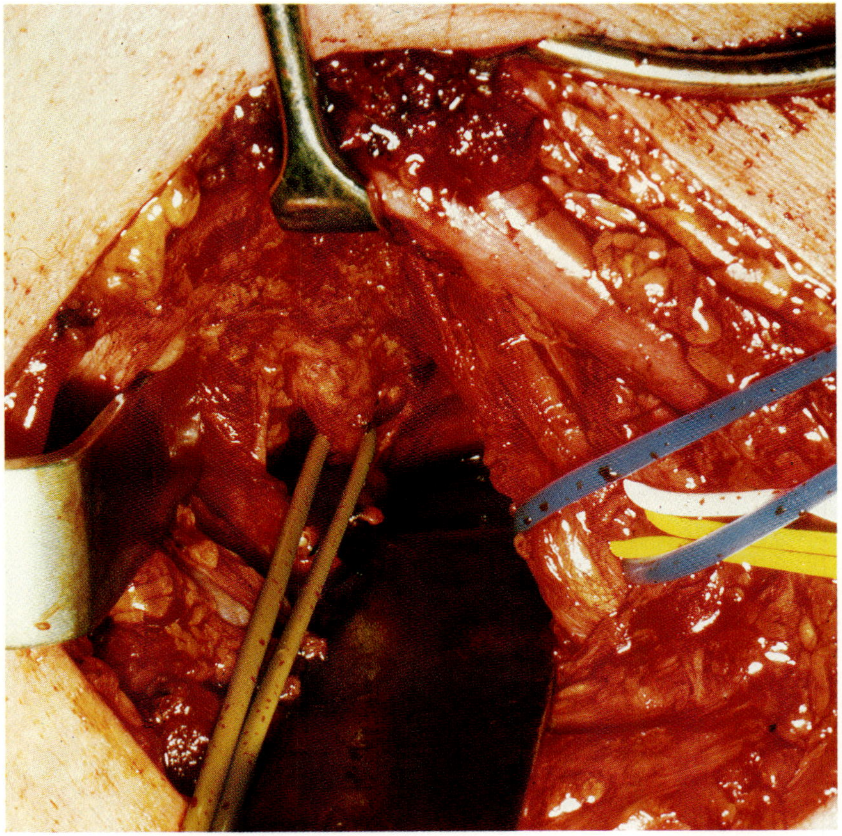

25 Ruptured Sibson's fascia to open the posterior mediastinum. Sibson's fascia is ruptured with a finger and a space is formed in the posterior mediastinum to the level of the third and fourth ribs. A long, narrow-bladed retractor, or narrow malleable copper retractor is used to hold the pleura downwards and laterally. Slings have been placed around the three trunks of the brachial plexus.

26 Exposure of the stellate ganglion. The stellate ganglion – combination of the inferior cervical and the first thoracic ganglion – is identified on the neck of the first rib by finger palpation. It is then carefully exposed with long scissors and forceps dissection. The sympathetic trunk below the ganglion is dissected and a sling passed around it for easy identification during dissection, and as a simple retractor.

27

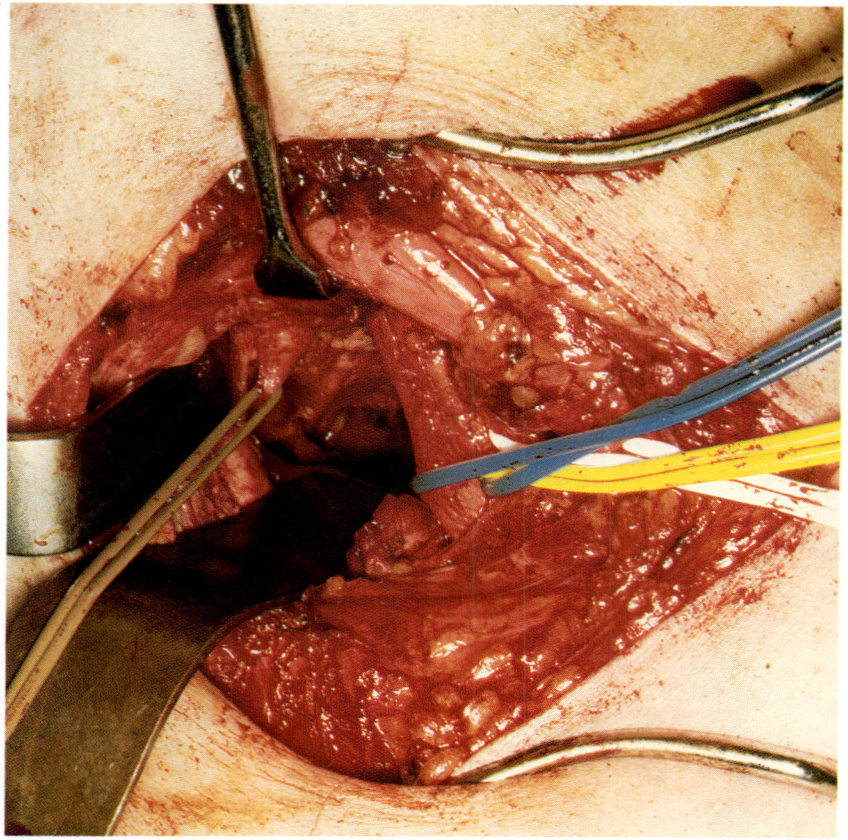

28

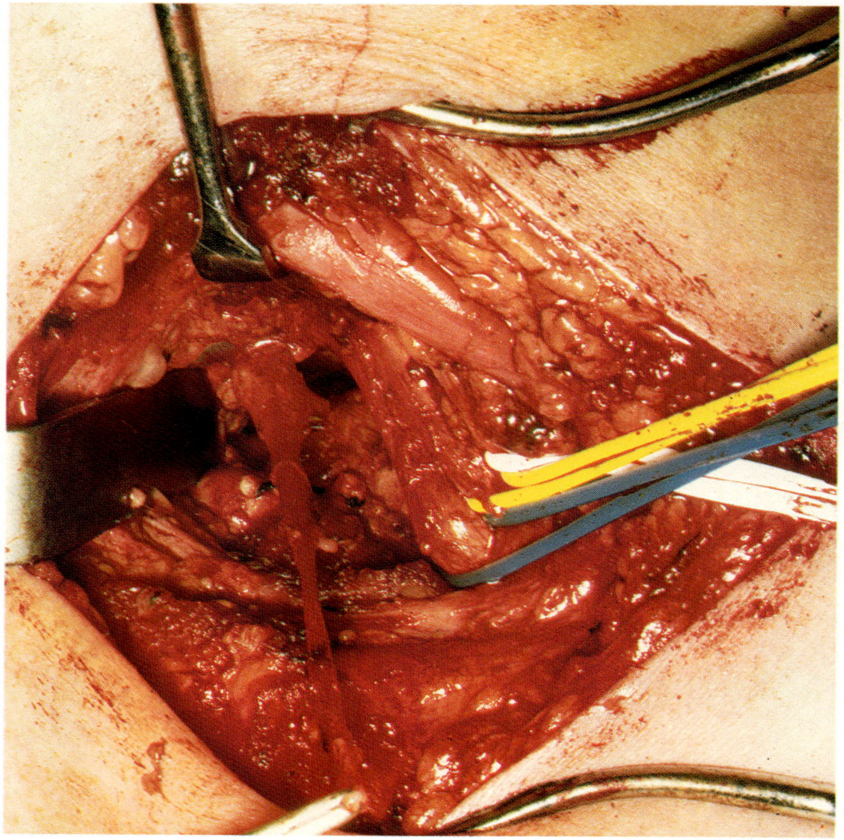

27 Dissection of the sympathetic chain. Well-focused overhead light, or a cavity light, is essential at this stage to identify the second and third ganglia with certainty, as well as to avoid damage to intercostal vessels. Minor venous bleeding is controlled by temporary pressure. More significant bleeding points from an intercostal artery or vein must be viewed by good light and adequate suction. The bleeding is controlled with long atraumatic forceps and application of diathermy coagulation. The white rami communicating with the second and third ganglia are divided carefully under direct vision and the sympathetic chain is cut below the third ganglion.

28 Division of the sympathetic chain below the third ganglion. The sympathetic chain has been divided below the third ganglion and brought to the surface. The lower pole of the stellate ganglion is divided and removed with the second and third ganglia.

29

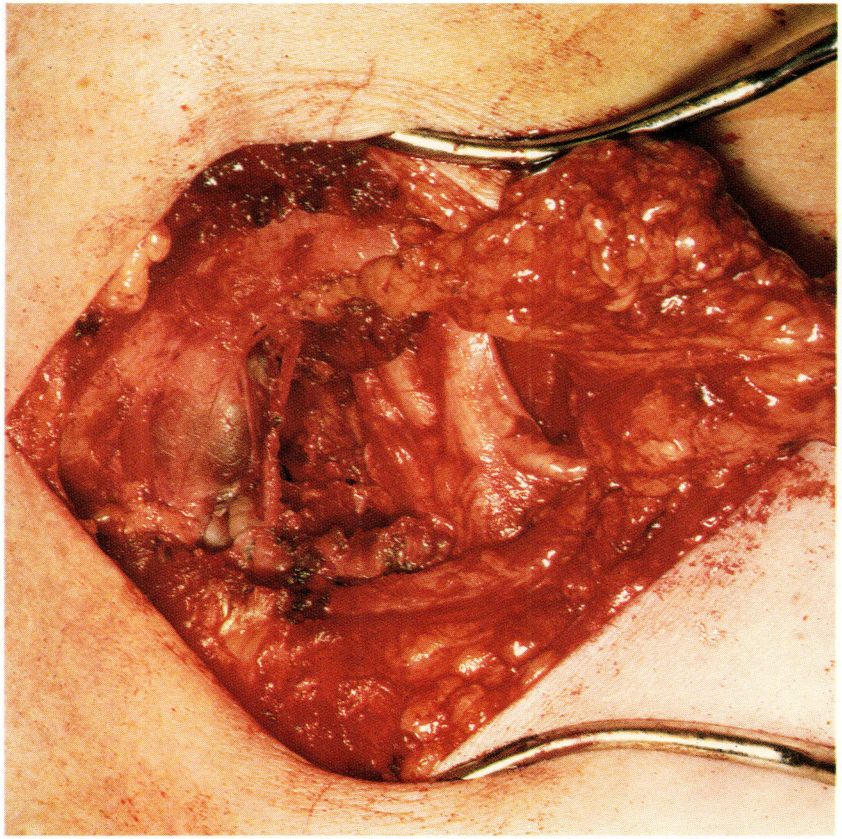

29 Final checking points. After removing the sympathetic chain the operation site is carefully checked for any bleeding that might cause a haematoma and scarring. The lungs are inflated to ensure that the pleura has not been damaged. The illustration shows the internal jugular vein, thoracic duct, phrenic nerve, and the brachial plexus. The pad of fat has been withdrawn from behind the omohyoid muscle.

30

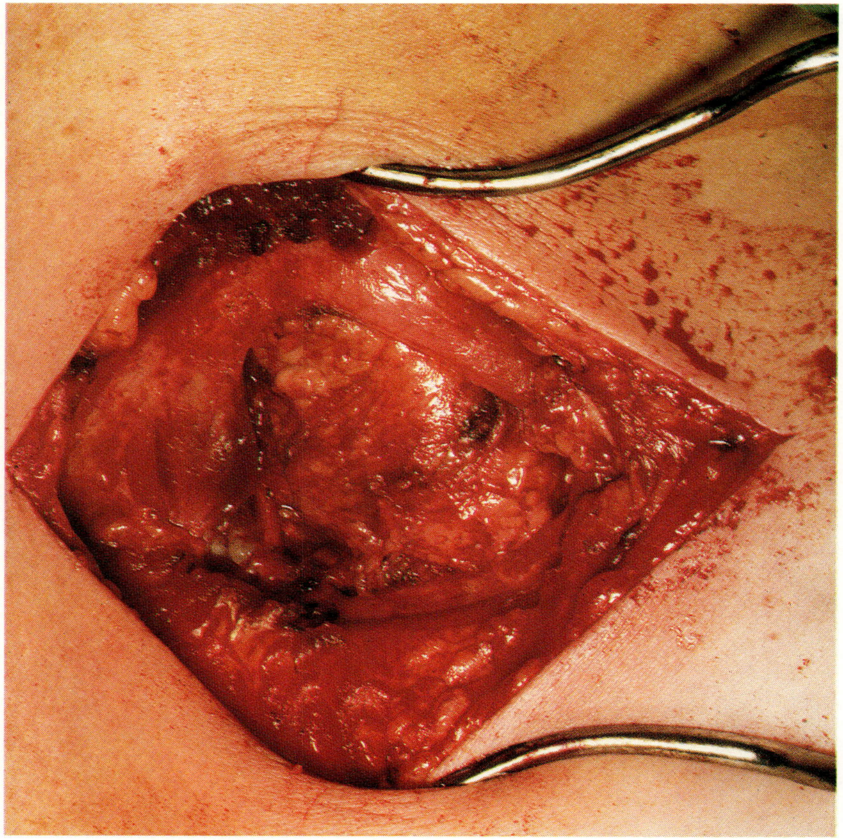

30 Replacement of the pad of fat. The pad of fat replaced over the brachial plexus and the residual cavity.

31 Closure. The clavicular head of the sternomastoid is resutured with 1.0 chromic catgut; the platysma layer is sutured with 3.0 plain catgut; the skin is closed with 3.0 subcuticular Dexon to ensure a fine scar. **Vacuum drainage is needed if haemostasis is not entirely complete.** Any puncture of the pleura demands an intrapleural vacuum drain for 24 hours. Complete expansion of the lung is checked radiologically before removing the drain.

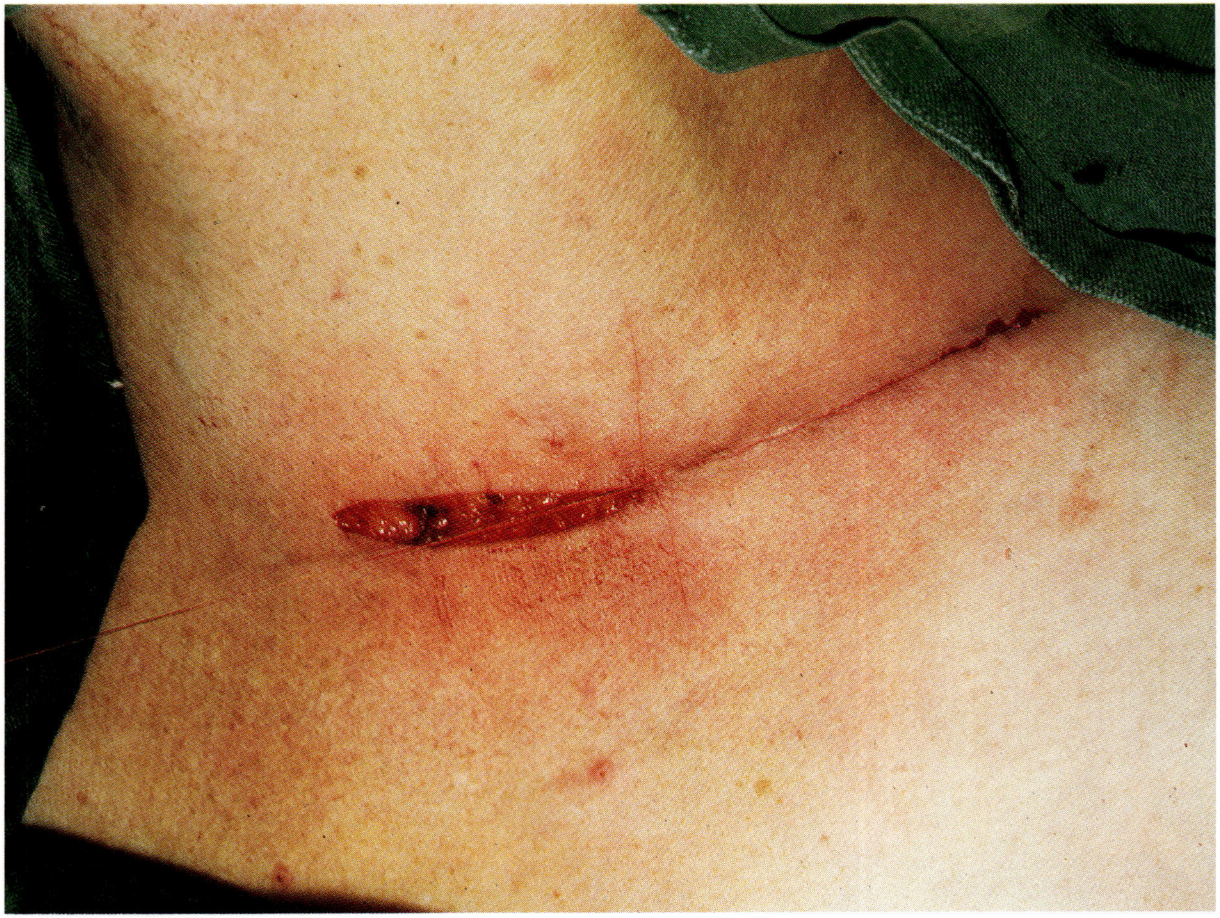

31

Excision of cervical rib and fascial bands

It is a truism to state that, whereas cervical ribs produce arterial problems, fascial bands cause neurological problems.

The cervical rib is not a true rib but rather an enlargement of the anterior root of the seventh cervical transverse process. It can exist as a separate bone varying in size between a tiny spicule of bone to a complete bridge of bone from the transverse process to the first rib, either immediately behind or just lateral to the scalene tubercle. When the rib is short or rudimentary, the gap to the first rib is completed by a fascial band.

Its clinical importance lies in the fact that the second part of the subclavian artery passes between the rib or fascial band and the scalenus anterior muscle. The C8 and T1 nerve roots pass over the rib or fascial band and can be stretched, irritated or damaged, giving rise to pain or atrophy of the small hand muscles. The arterial and neurological problems will be discussed separately.

Compression of the artery intermittently during exercise causes ischaemic symptoms as described in the introduction. The wall of the artery can be damaged with the formation of thrombus with or without the presence of atheroma. The classical post-stenotic aneurysm occurs at this site in the third part of the subclavian artery. Short[4] showed that when the rib is attached immediately behind the scalenus anterior muscle, the aneurysm will be fusiform in shape. When the cervical rib is attached lateral to the scalenus anterior, the artery forms two right-angles as it traverses the space and the increased turbulence produces a saccular aneurysm. Thrombosis within the artery or aneurysm can be an important source of distal emboli threatening the viability of finger, hand, or even forearm. **Distal emboli can occur suddenly with the danger of distal gangrene.** It must be realised that subclavian aneurysms are rarely palpable because they are situated behind the clavicle.

Should all cervical ribs be removed?

The operation is not without danger to the friable subclavian artery and brachial plexus. Damage to the brachial plexus can produce intractable postoperative pain, loss of sensation and muscle power.

The indications for excising a cervical rib are:

1 The presence of distal emboli.
2 The presence of an aneurysm diagnosed clinically or on angiography.
3 Pain and/or pallor incompatible with daily work.
4 Total occlusion of the artery in active abduction and external rotation.
5 The presence of a persistent bruit over the artery in any position of the arm.

Additional procedures for excising a saccular aneurysm and inserting a vein graft may be necessary as well as a cervicodorsal sympathectomy to promote healing of distal focal necrosis. Thrombectomy will suffice when there is no aneurysm and thrombus has formed on damaged endothelium an atheromatous plaque or a fusiform aneurysm.

Obstruction of the subclavian artery from other causes must be mentioned here because they need the same exposure.

1 Thrombosis from atheroma. If the first part of the subclavian artery is affected, the Steal syndrome occurs, but in the second part it produces only a local effect.
2 Thrombosis after direct or blunt injury to the artery. Thrombosis can also occur after a stretch injury, such as hyperabduction of the arm,
3 Thrombosis may follow radiotherapy for pulmonary or breast tumours.

32
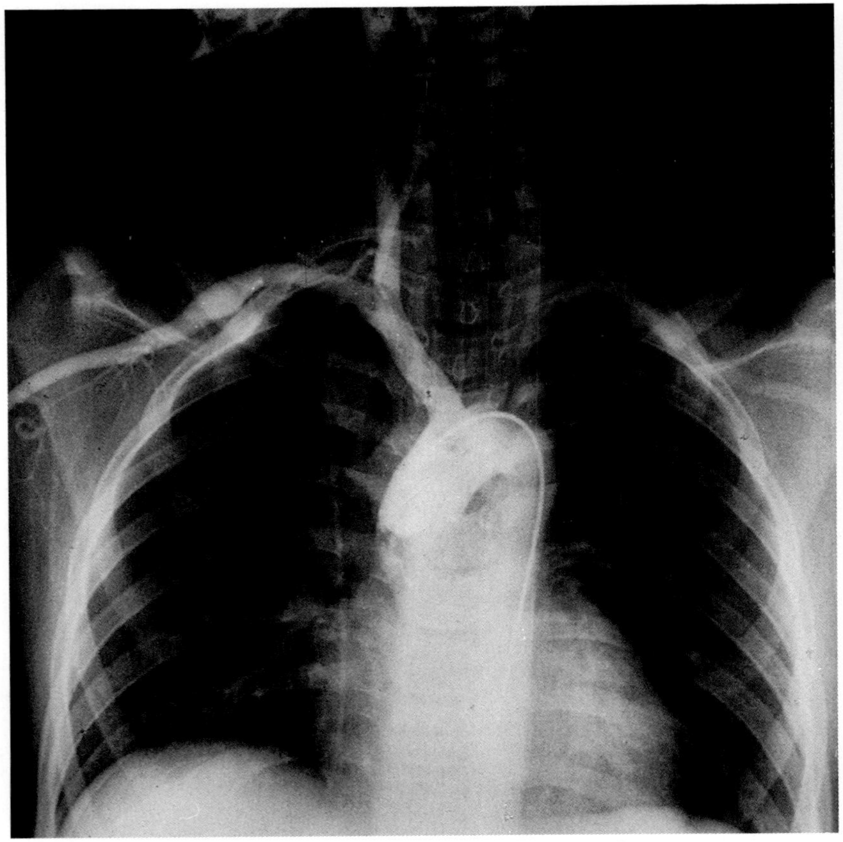

33
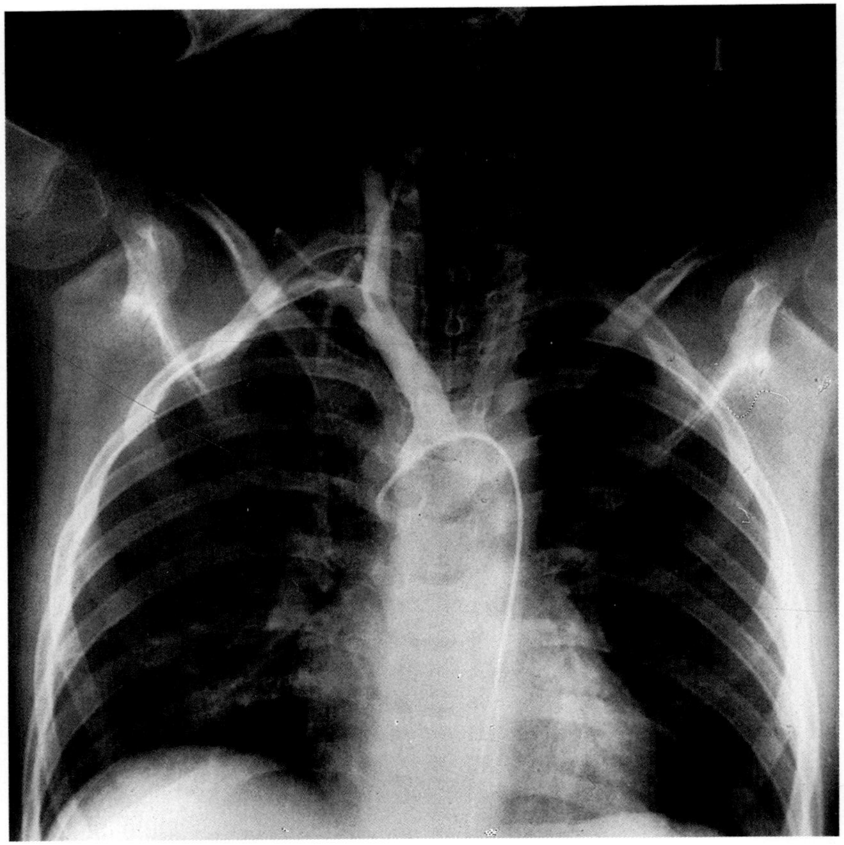

32 Cervical rib and arteriogram. Xray showing a large cervical rib with arteriogram showing a normal calibre subclavian artery with the arm in adduction.

33 Cervical rib and angiogram in abduction. Arteriogram with the arm in abduction shows total obstruction of the artery between the clavicle and the first and cervical rib.

34 Poststenotic dilatation of the subclavian artery. Operation picture of the subclavian artery showing fusiform dilatation.

34

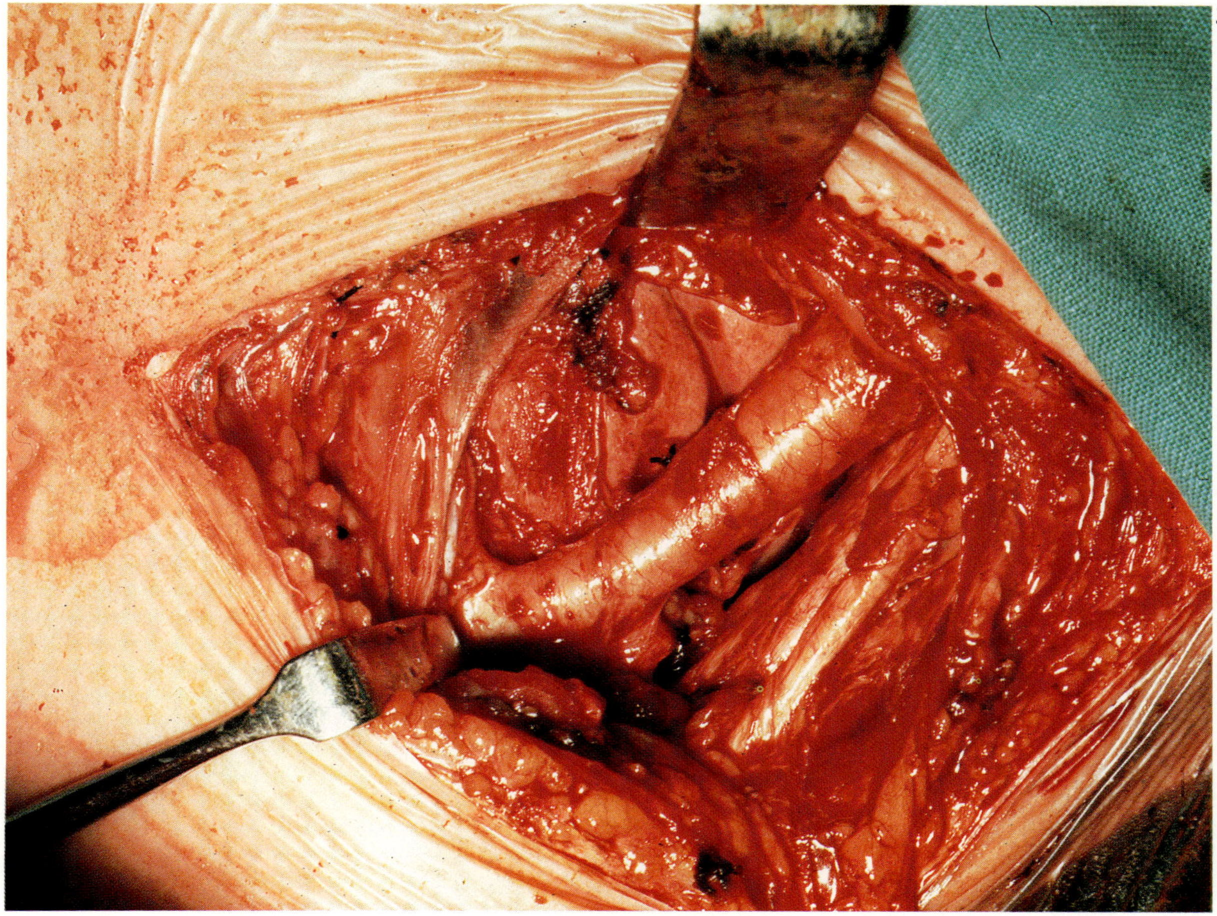

35 Excised cervical rib. Large bulky cervical rib removed and symptoms relieved.

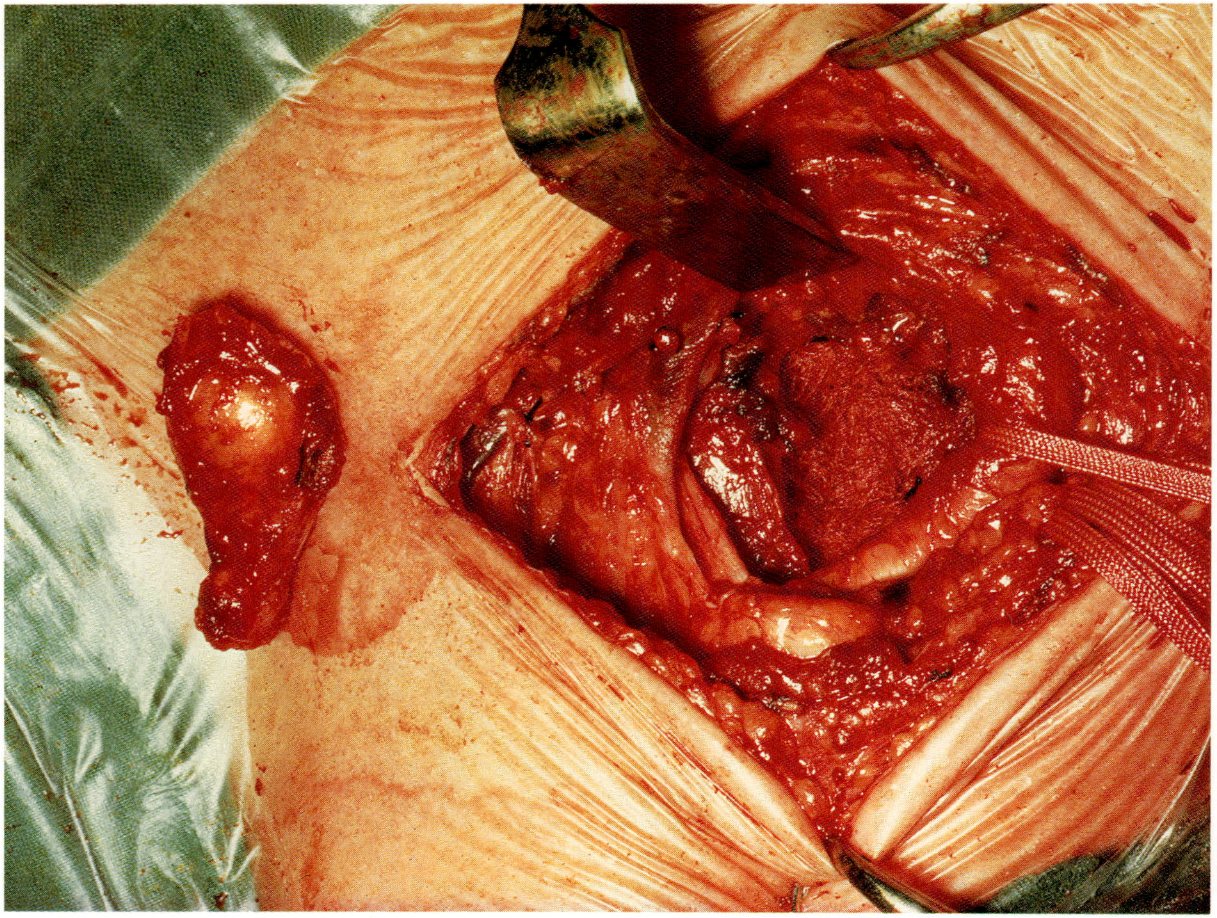
35

36 Cervical rib and beaked transverse process. Xray showing large left-sided cervical rib and a right beaked C7 transverse process.

36

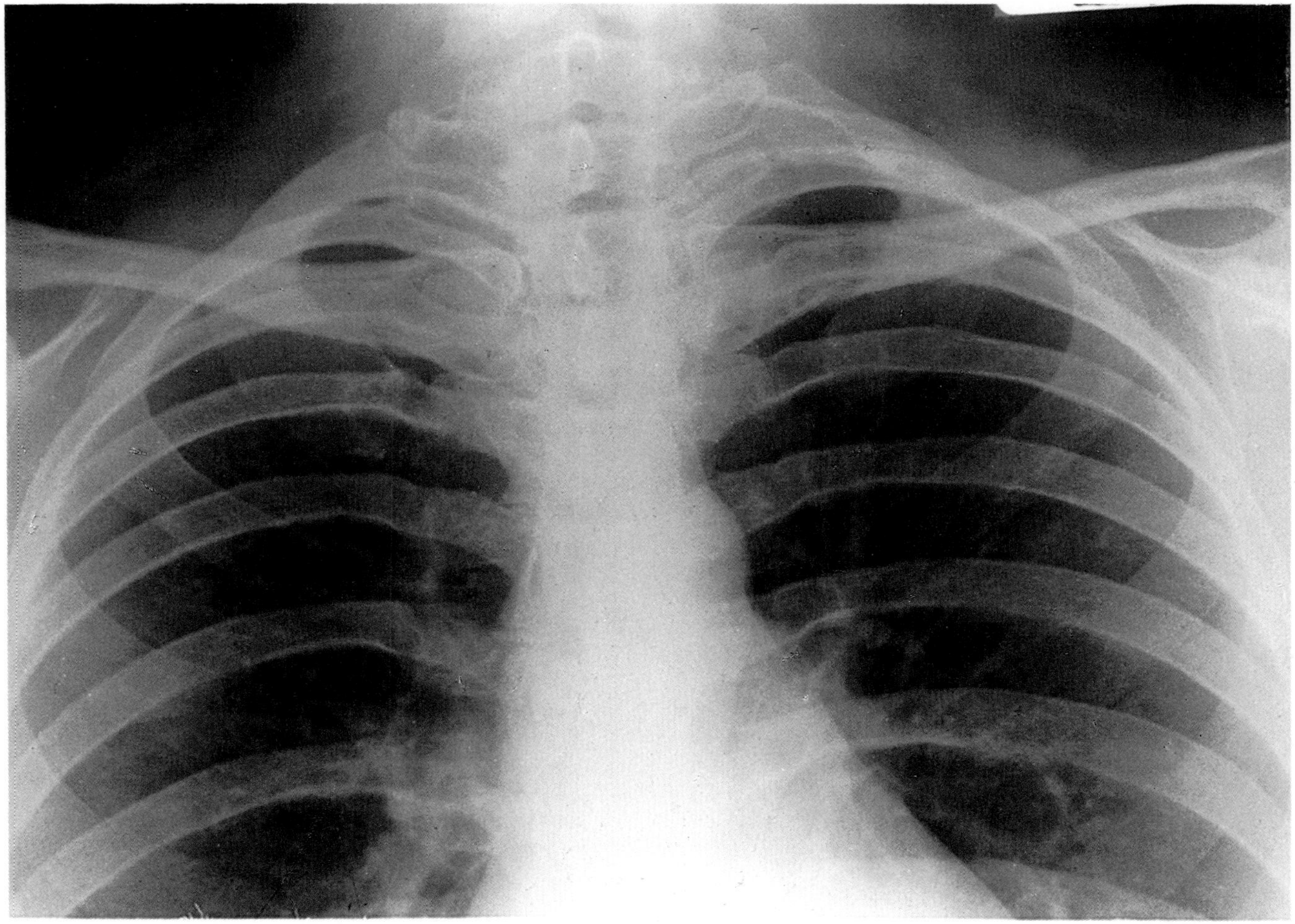

37

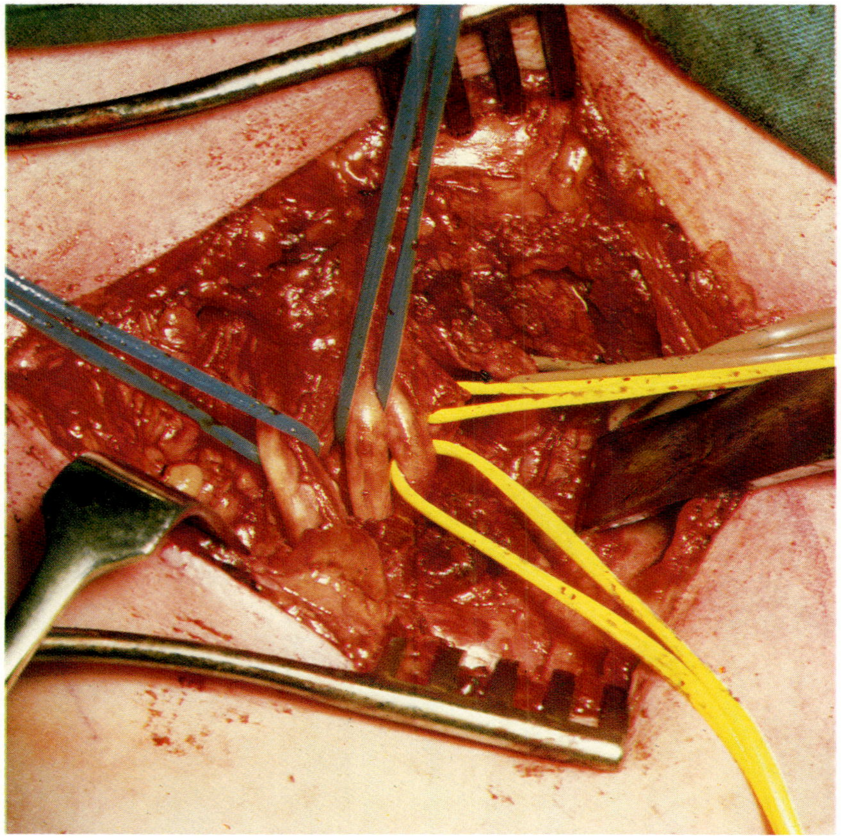

38

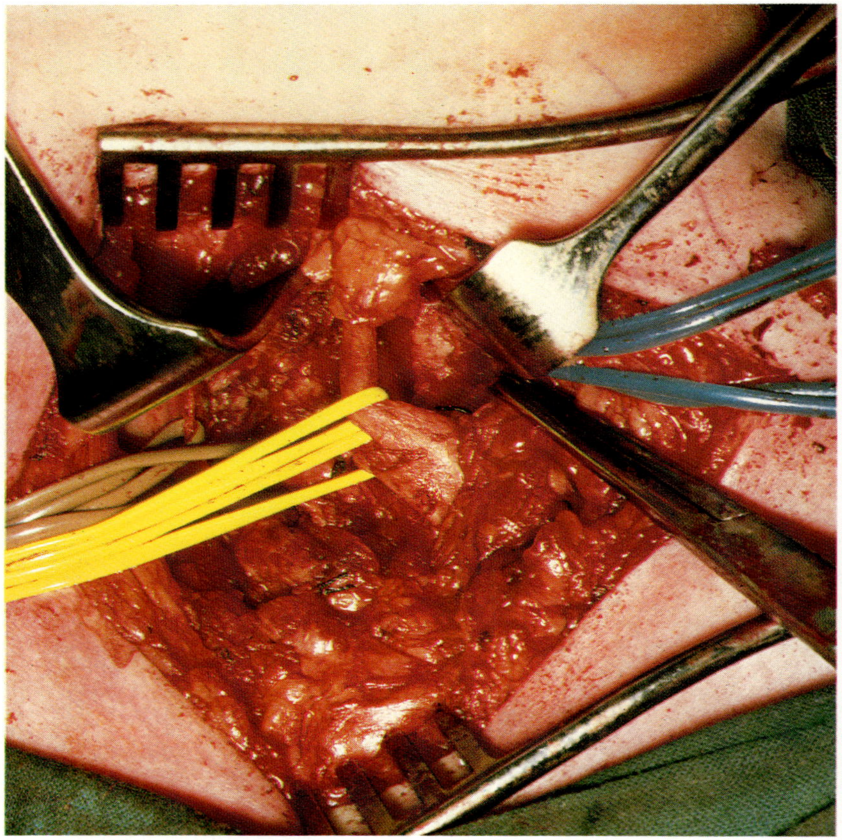

37 Identification of nerve roots. The C5,6,7,8, and T1 roots of the plexus are identified. The connective tissue between the roots is carefully divided and the roots, as well as the upper, middle, and lower trunks separated. Slings are passed around individual roots or trunks, so that they can be held apart without tension. Yellow slings shown around C5,6, and 7, and blue slings around C8 and T1 roots.

38 Exposure of the upper end of the cervical rib. Roots C8 and T1 are separated from C7, and the cervical rib is found in the gap surrounded by muscle fibres of the scalenus medius muscle. The rib is easily palpated and easily seen after dividing surrounding muscle fibres.

39 Division of the cervical rib. The muscle fibres are cut away from the rib which is then divided with straight bone cutters. The upper portion is dissected from its muscle bed and removed with rongeurs to its attachment to the transverse process of the seventh cervical vertebra.

39

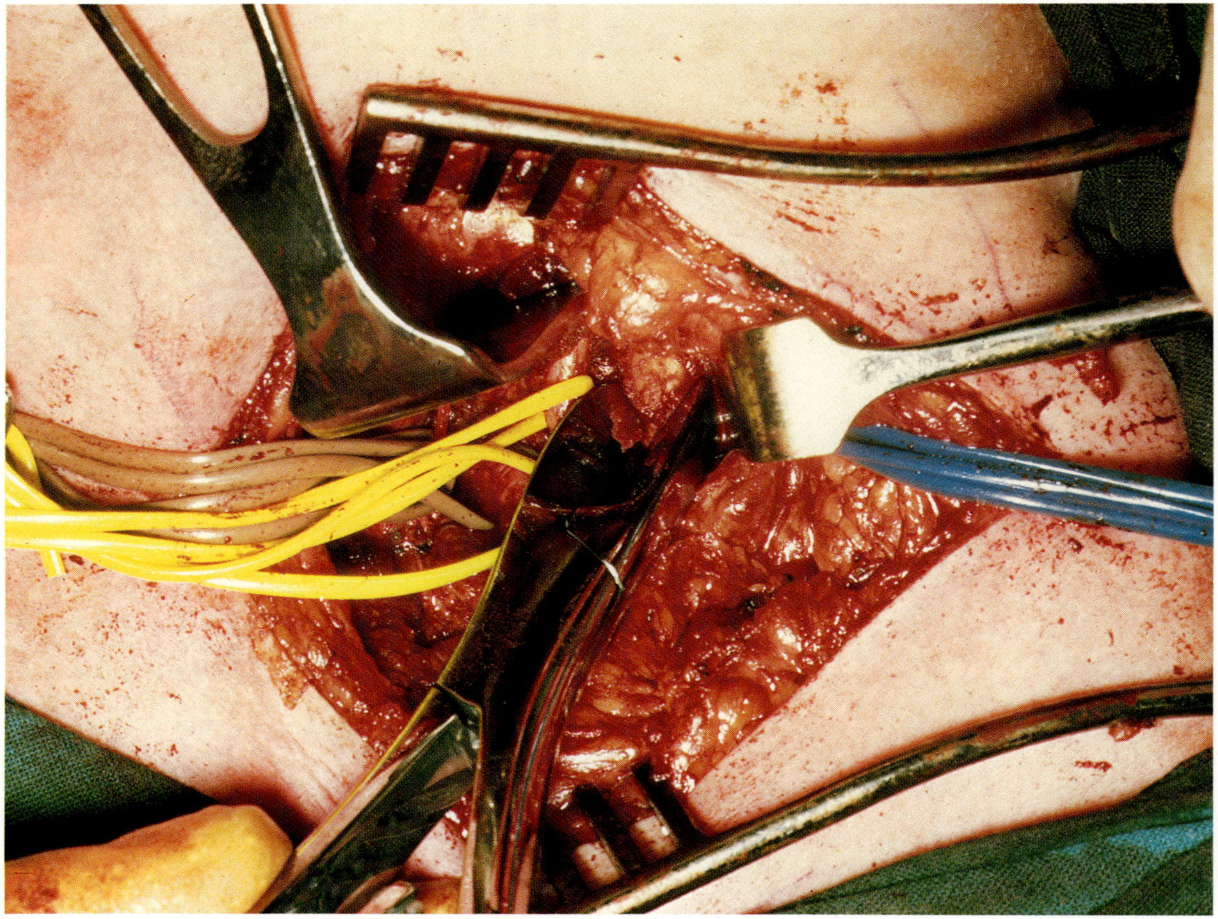

40 Post-excision space. Gap between C7–C8 after removal of the upper end of the cervical rib.

40

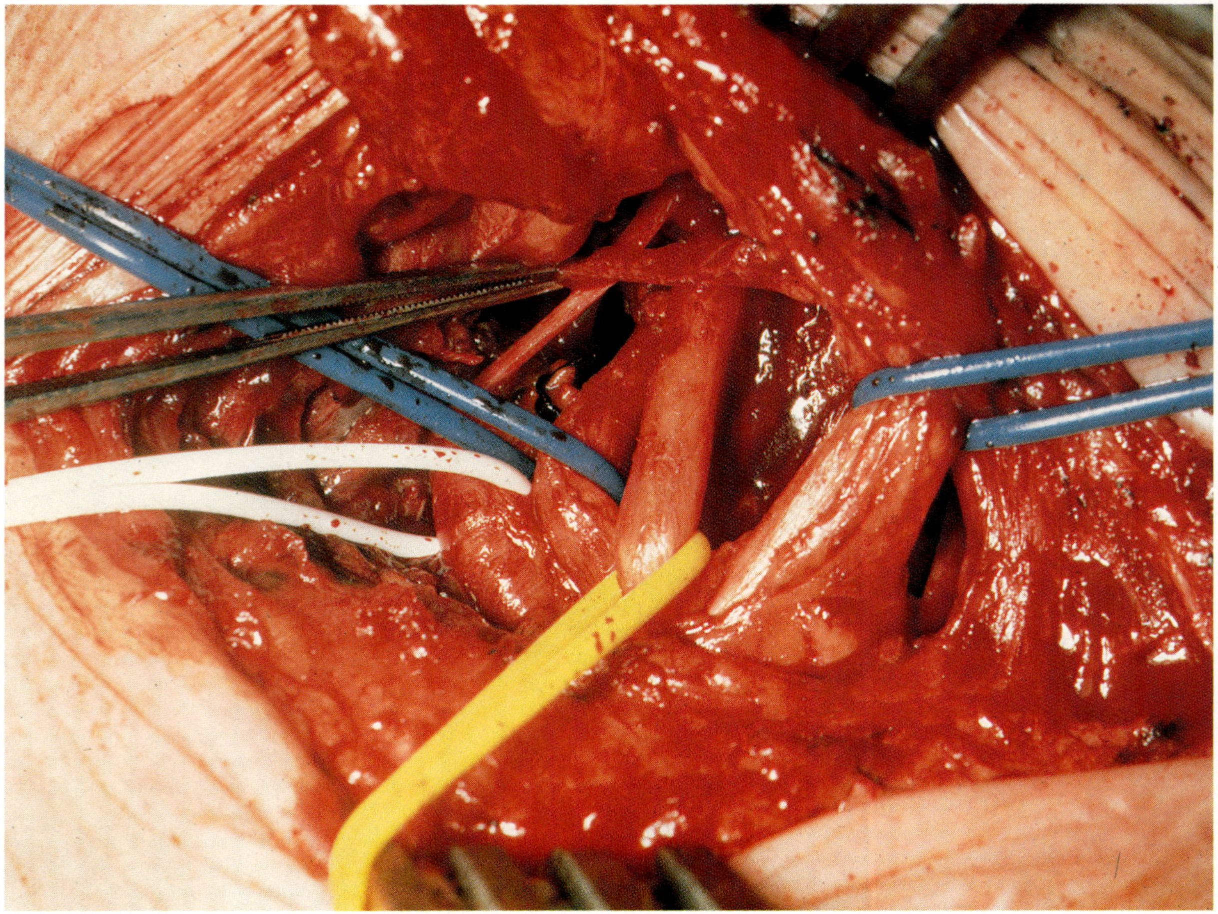

41

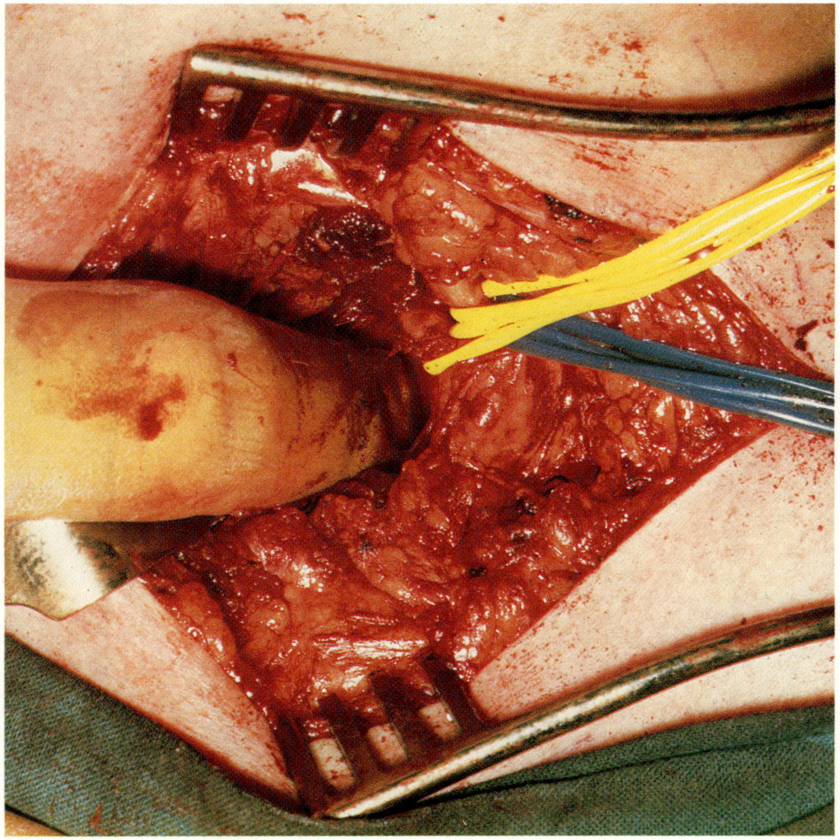

42

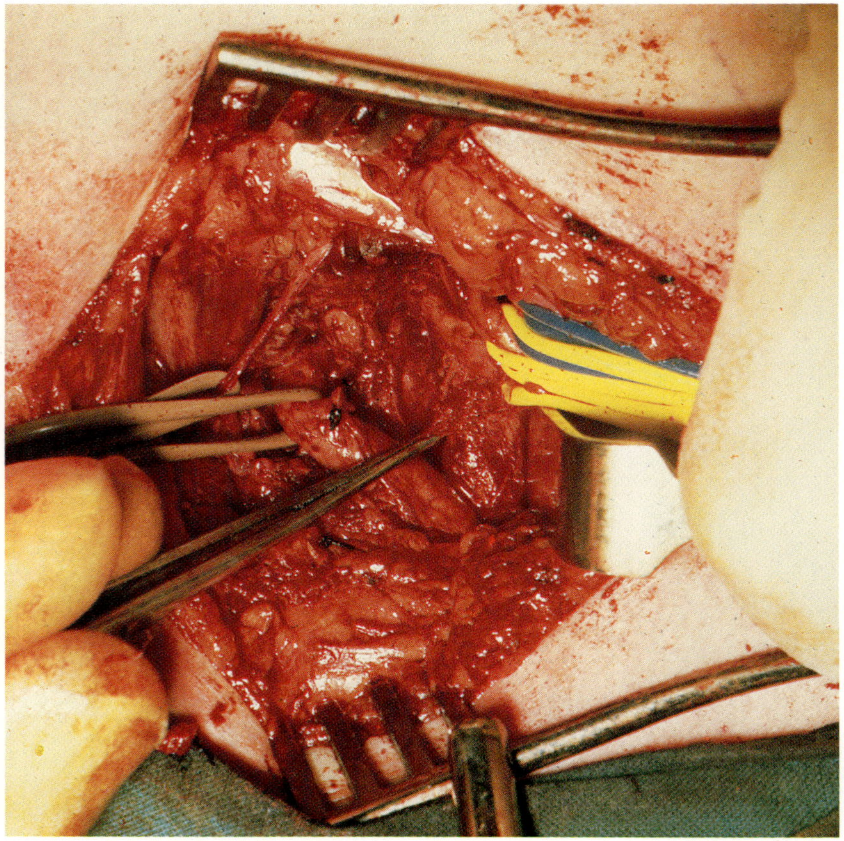

41 and 42 Exposure of the lower end of the cervical rib. The lower portion is then palpated and exposed, medial to the plexus and behind the subclavian artery.

43

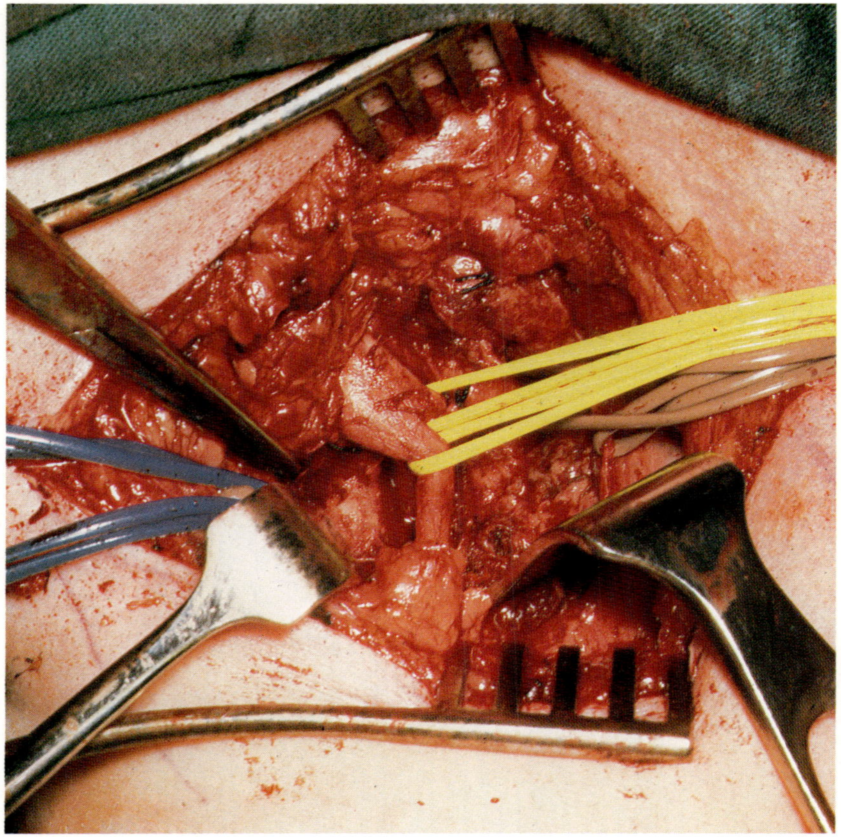

44

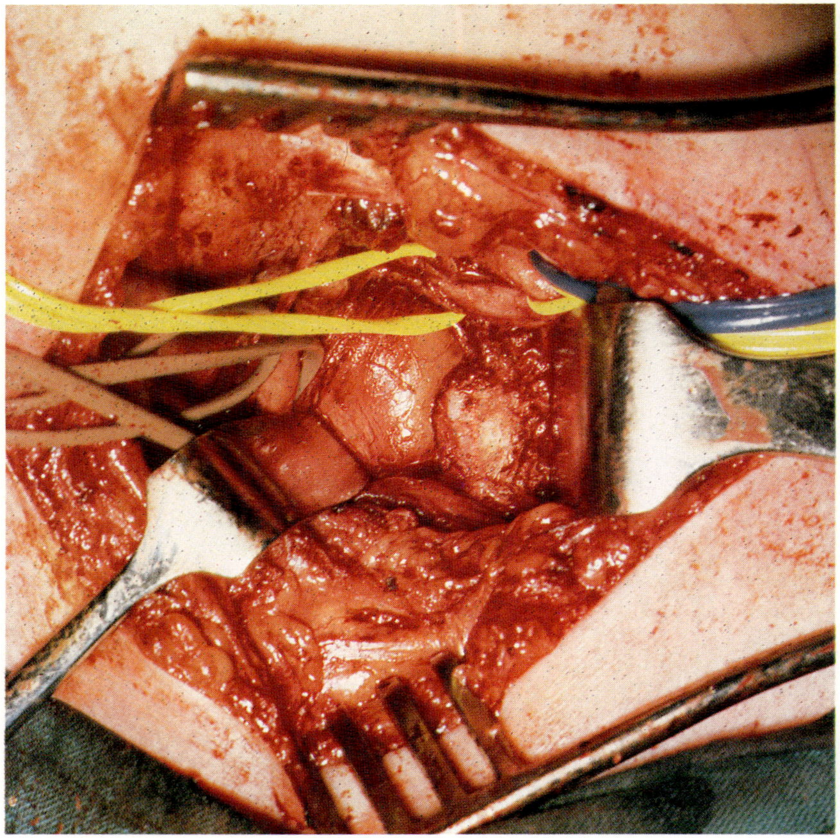

43 Dissection of the lower end of the cervical rib. The rib is separated from surrounding muscle by sharp dissection with a knife and scissors.

44 Lower end exposed attached to the first rib. When isolated to its lower attachment to the first rib it is detached by a knife, bone cutter or chisel, depending on whether the attachment is fibrous, a false joint or an irregular bony union.

45 Excised cervical rib. Cervical rib with large lower end which formed a false joint with the first rib.

45

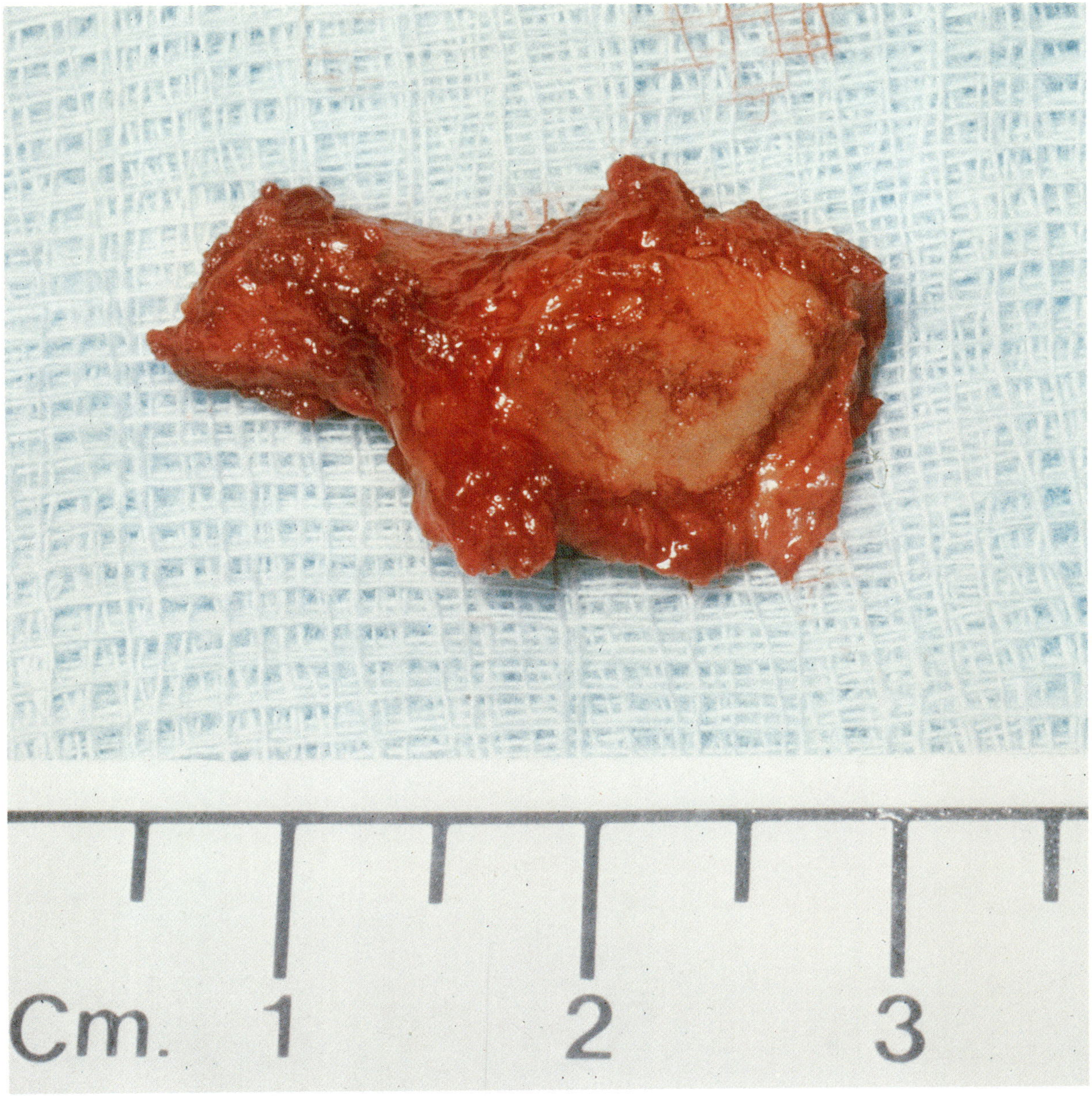

46

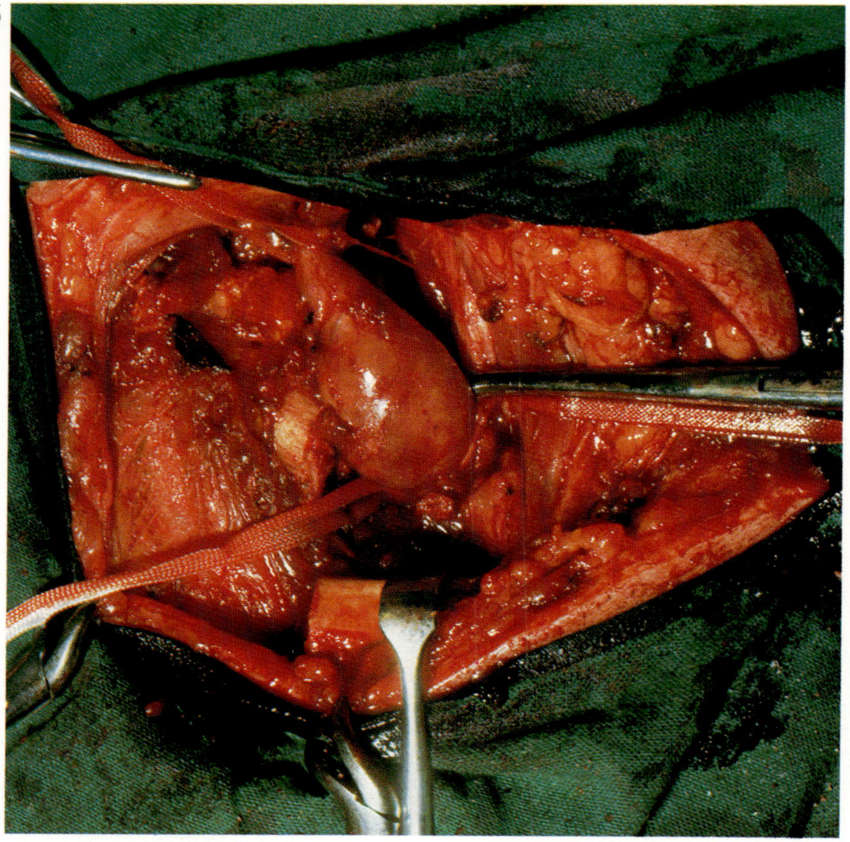

47

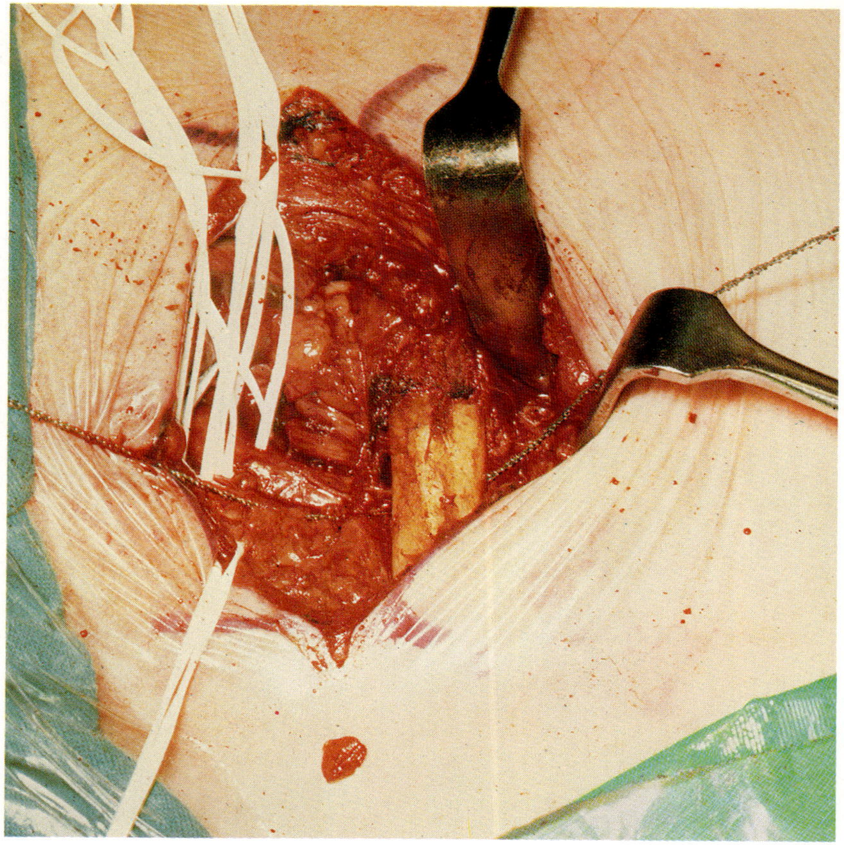

46 Subclavian aneurysm. A coinciding subclavian aneurysm may need resection at the same time. The aneurysm is exposed completely by dividing the clavicle at the junction of its middle and outer thirds. This allows clamping of the subclavian and axillary arteries and the excision of the aneurysm.

47 Division of the clavicle. The periosteum is stripped off the bone and a Gigli saw passed sub-periosteally around the clavicle. The bone is then divided without risk of injury to the local blood vessels or nerves.

48 Vein graft replacement. A reversed saphenous vein graft is inserted to bridge the gap.

48

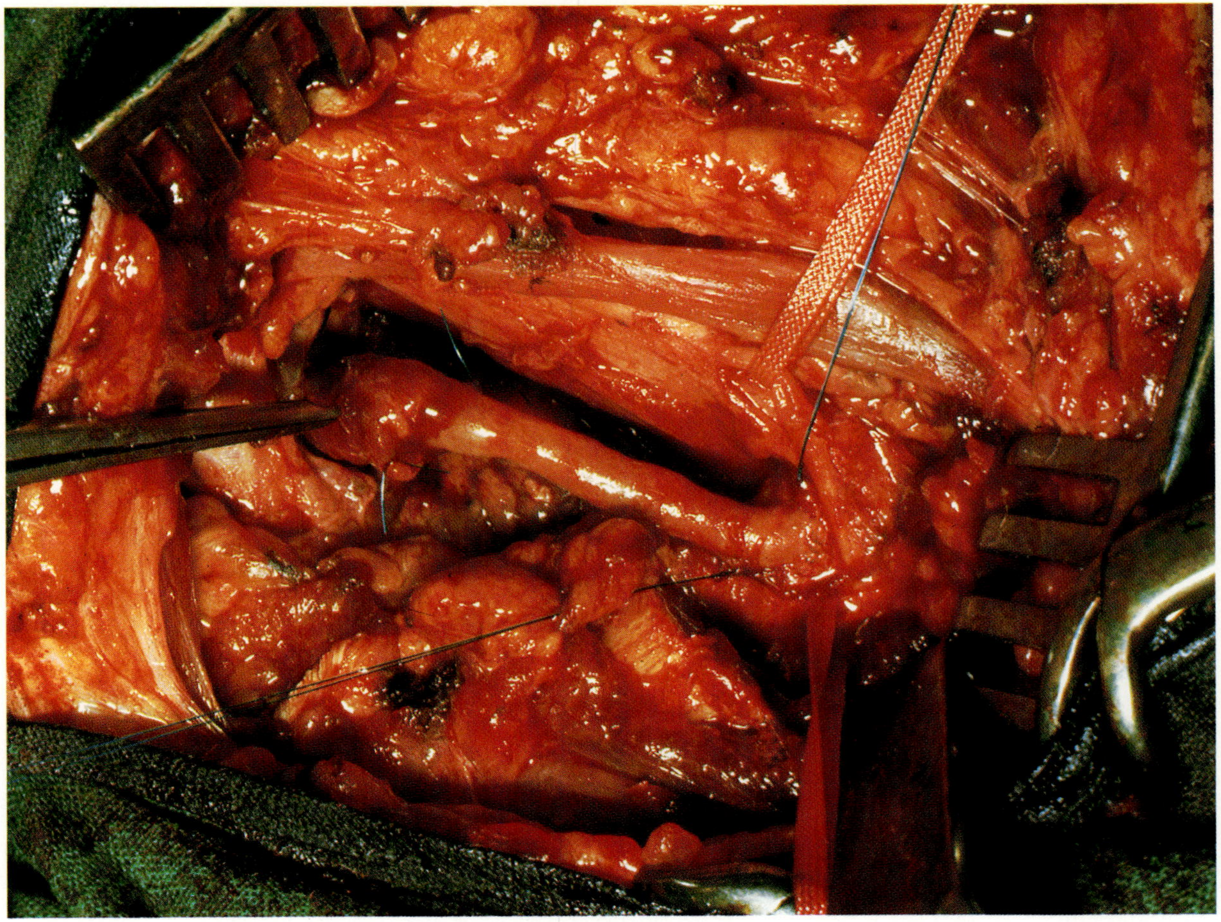

49

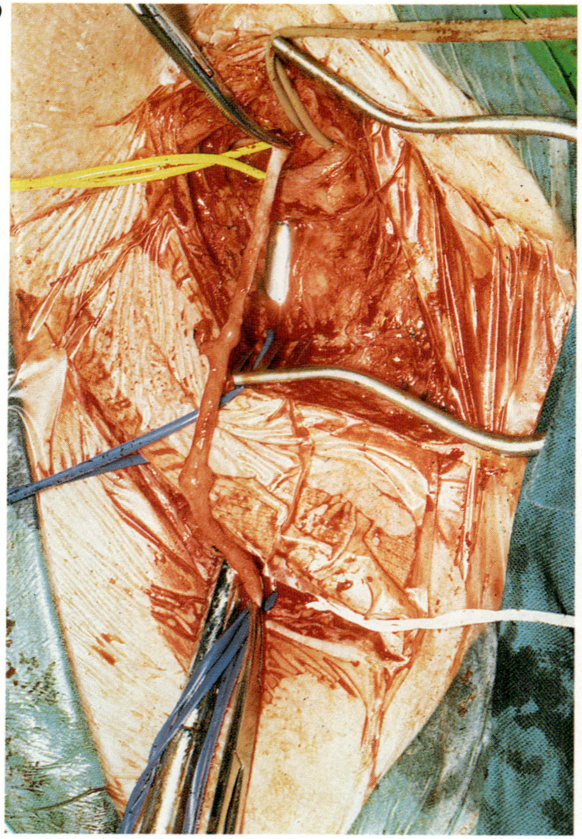

50

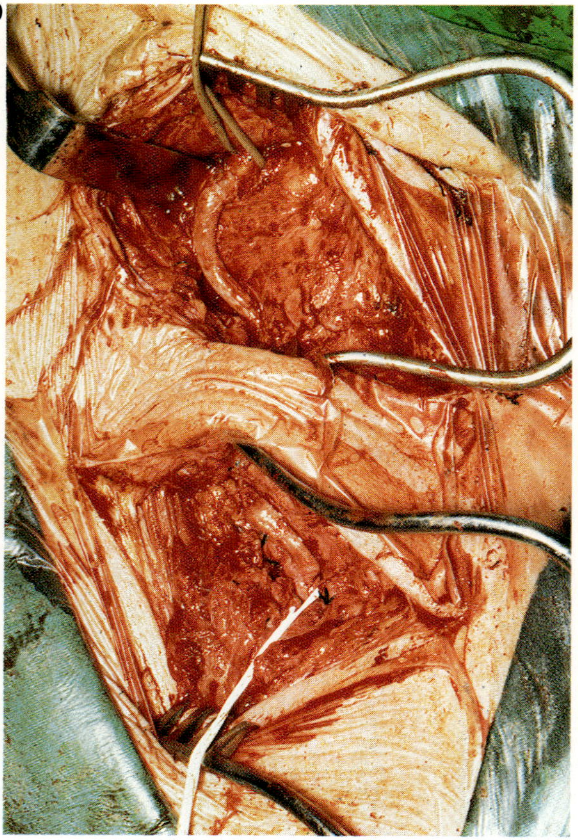

51

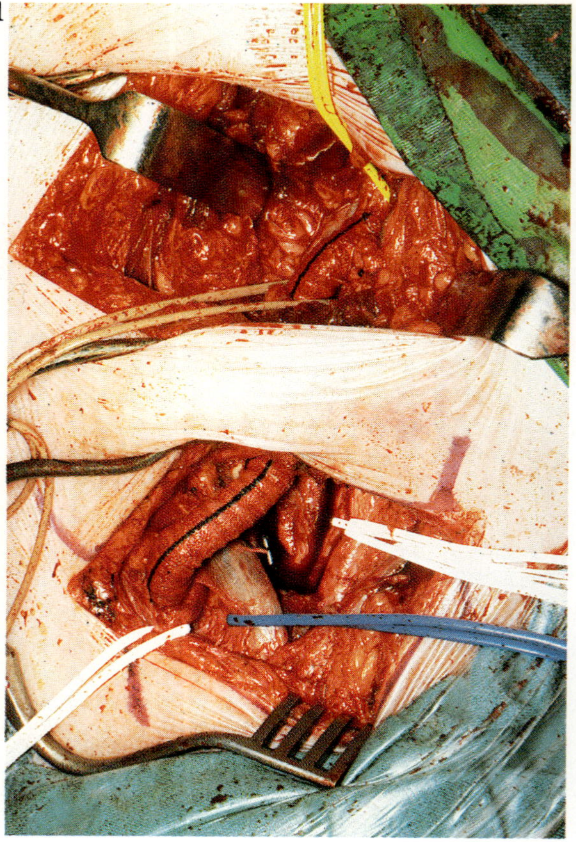

49 Subclavian – axillary vein graft. An alternative procedure is to expose the axillary artery below the clavicle, and the graft passed behind the clavicle for anastomosis to the axillary artery. Saphenous vein – dilated with saline – reversed and measured for correct length. A blunt dilator is passed from below upwards to form a channel for insertion of the vein graft.

50 Vein graft in position behind the clavicle. A retroclavicular reversed saphenous vein graft to by-pass the subclavian artery obstruction caused through hyperabduction injury.

51 Carotid–axillary bypass graft. Synthetic Dacron bypass graft from the common carotid artery to the axillary artery for post-irradiation thrombosis of the subclavian artery. A section of the clavicle was removed for safe exposure. A similar graft from the common carotid to the subclavian artery is used to correct the Steal syndrome.

Excision of fascial bands

Fascial bands are recognised in three anatomical sites:

1 In the same position as a cervical rib. It passes from a rudimentary rib or a beaked transverse process of the seventh cervical vertebra to the first rib behind the scalene tubercle.

2 It exists as, or indistinguishable from, the knife-like medial edge of the scalenus medius muscle.

3 It may be a short, tight fibrous band in the posteromedial part of Sibson's fascia. It passes from the C7 transverse process to the posterior part of the first rib just distal to its neck. This band is probably a remnant of the scalenus pleuralis, itself a part of the scalenus medius muscle.

In all the situations, the C8 and T1 nerve roots can be stretched over the band, irritated, trapped or damaged by recurring pressure against the sharp edges. The fascial bands are primarily associated with neurological symptoms of pain, paraesthesia or numbness in the ulnar distribution and/or motor weakness as described in the introduction. The bands can of course give rise to arterial problems in the same way as a cervical rib can, on occasions, cause neurological damage.

Operations for neurological symptoms can be disappointing and symptoms persist or can be aggravated. Not only are fascial bands and cervical ribs responsible for symptoms, but the neck of the first rib can also affect the T1 root and add to the stretching and nerve irritation. Because of this, I always fully decompress the C8–T1 roots by removing, not only the cervical rib or fascial band, but also the first rib where neurological symptoms predominate. The long-term results are much better and a second more difficult and less satisfactory operation avoided.

To achieve removal of the first rib together with a cervical rib or fascial band, supraclavicular and infraclavicular exposures are used.

52

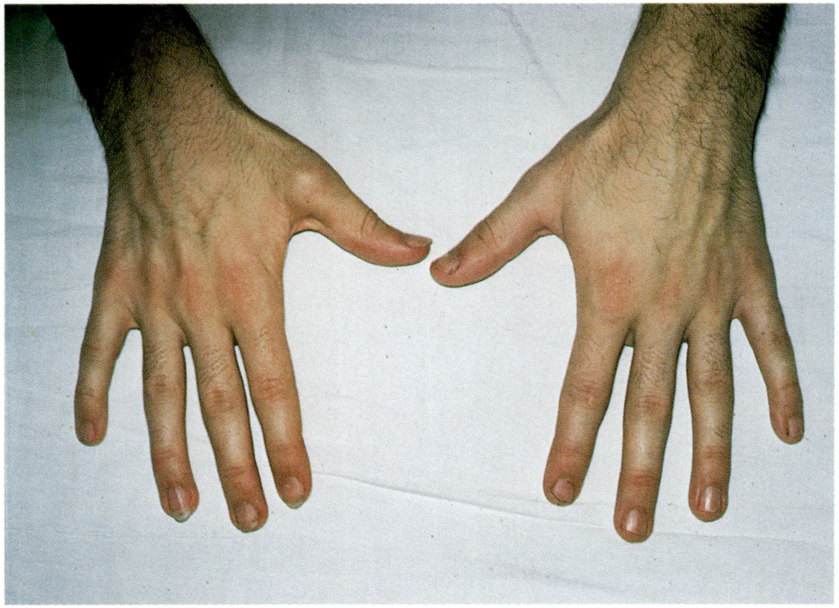

53

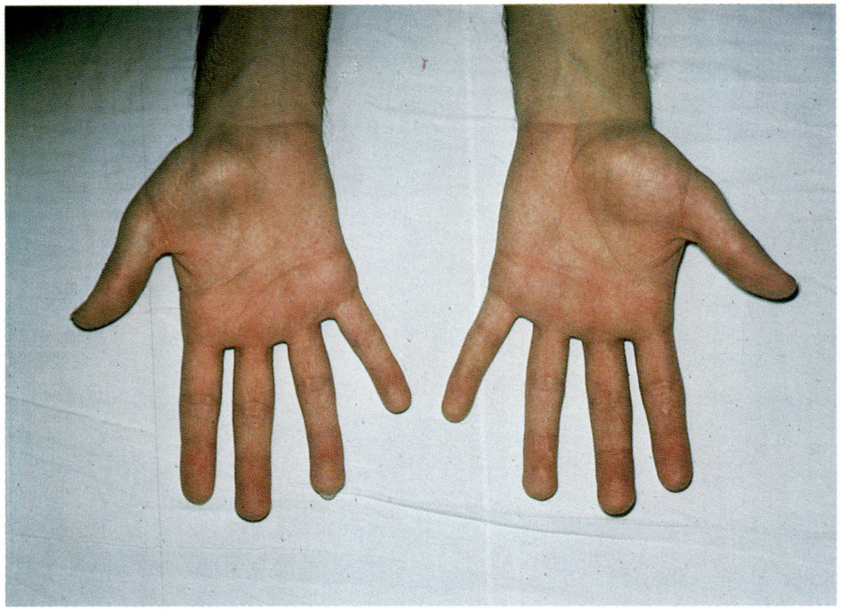

52 Dorsal view of hand with muscle atrophy. Dorsal view of the hands with wasting of the interossei muscles and the adductor pollicis between the thumb and the index finger.

53 Palmar view of hand with muscle atrophy. Photograph of the hands of a 19-year-old male with progressive weakness and muscle atrophy of the right hand. In the palmar view note the wasting of the thenar eminence caused by atrophy of the adductor pollicis.

54 Supraclavicular stage of decompression C8–T1 nerve roots. The operation is planned to remove a suspected fascial band and also remove the first rib to fully decompress C8 and T1 nerve roots.

Supraclavicular and infraclavicular incisions and exposures are used.

The supraclavicular exposure is carried out as in **1** to **18.**

The roots of the brachial plexus are separated and held on individual slings. Particular attention is paid to C8 and T1 roots and T1 must be exposed in relation to the neck of the rib.

Fascial bands are looked for in the three primary sites:

1 Between C7 and C8, in the presence of a beaked transverse process of the seventh cervical vertebra or a rudimentary cervical rib.

2 Behind and medial to the plexus for the sharp band in the medial edge of scalenus medius.

3 In the posterior part of Sibson's fascia as a short usually tough band from the C7 transverse process to just beyond the neck or angle of the first rib. Both C8 and T1 roots are trapped in a tight triangle between the band, the first rib, and the seventh cervical transverse process.

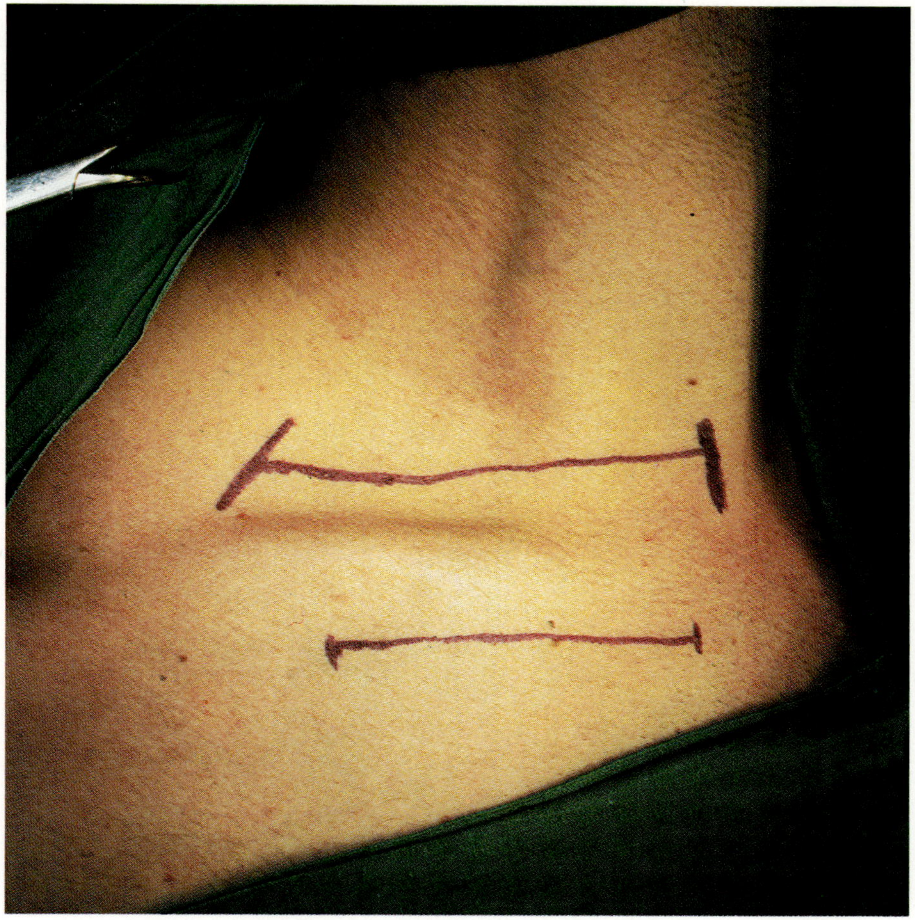

54

55 Fascial band in Sibson's fascia. Sibson's fascia is cleared and fibrous band isolated posteriorly in Sibson's fascia and trapping C8 and T1 roots, the C7 transverse process and the first rib.

55

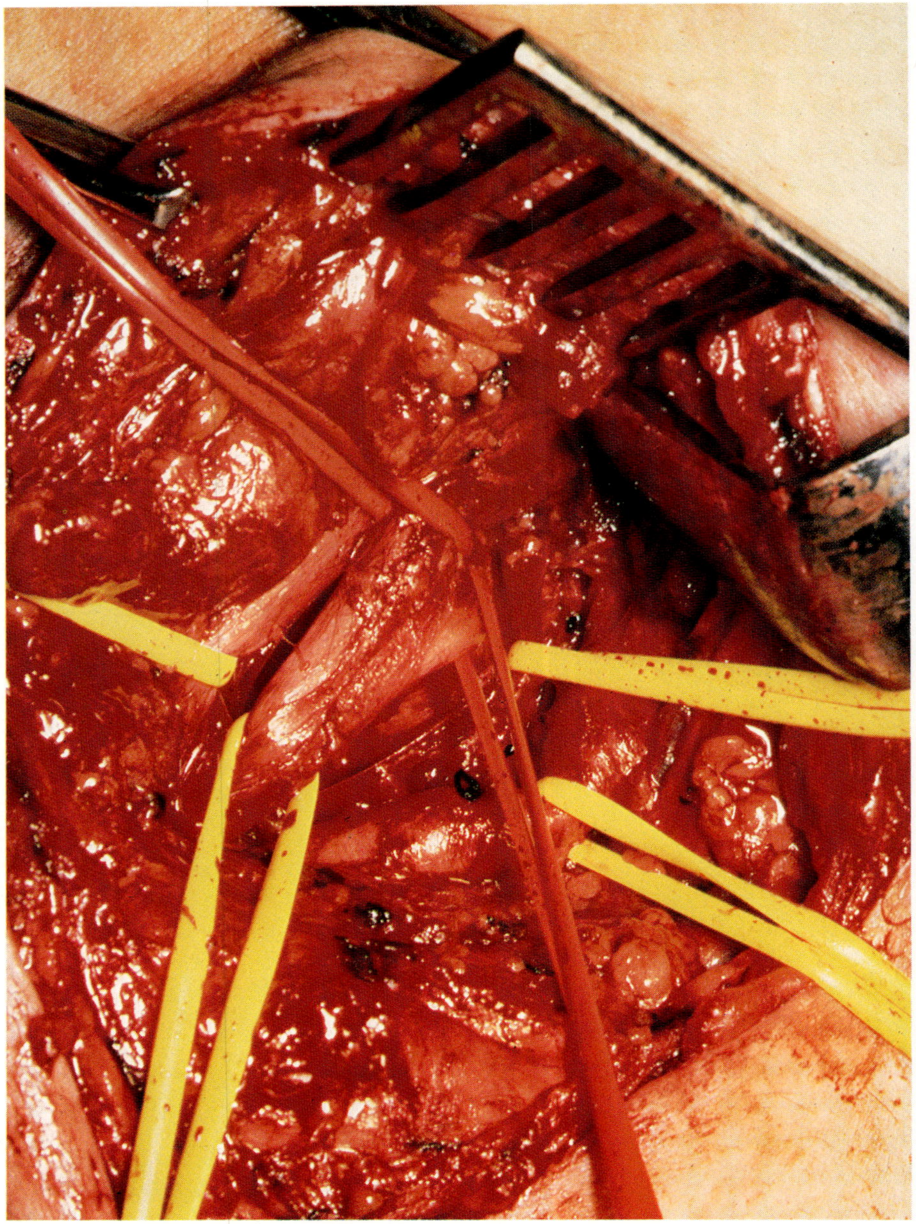

56 Close-up view of fascial band. A close view of the tough fascial band which is totally excised.

56

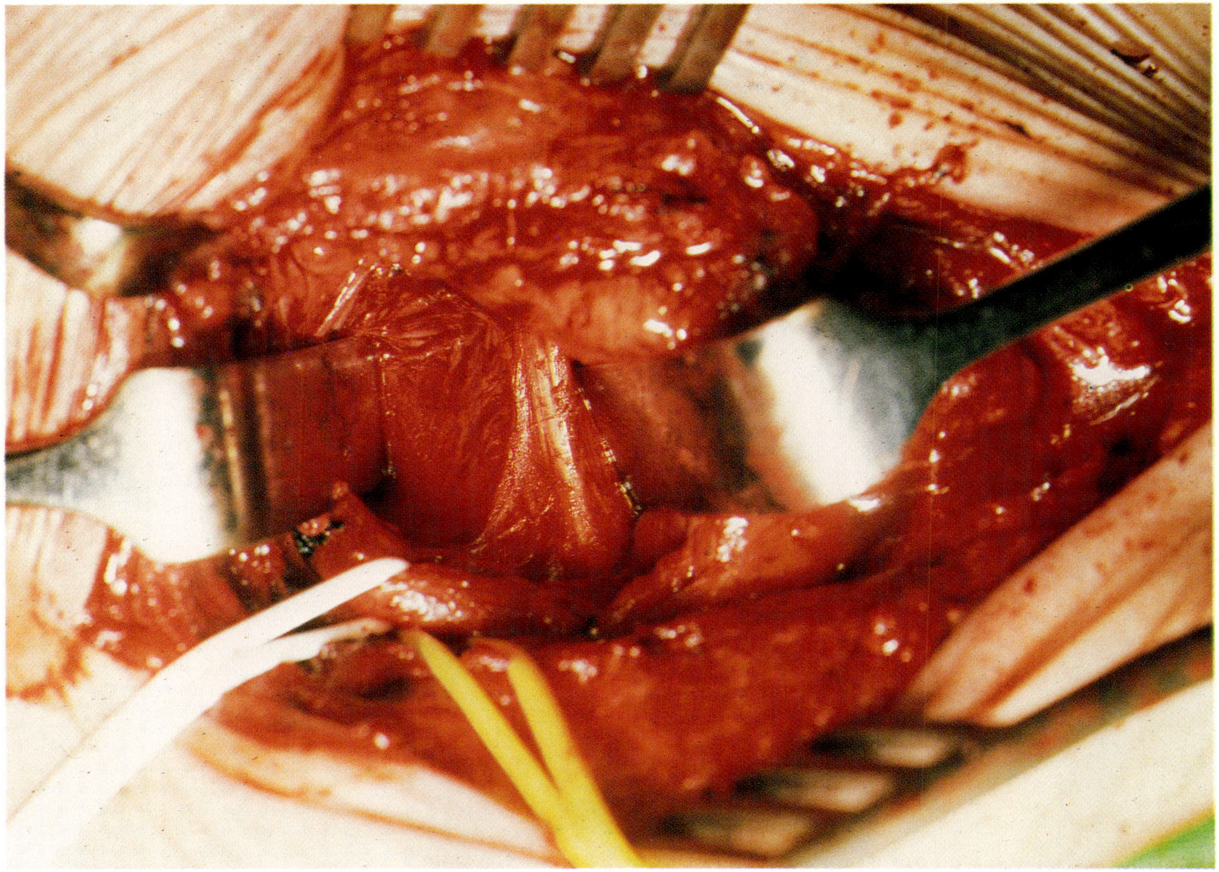

57

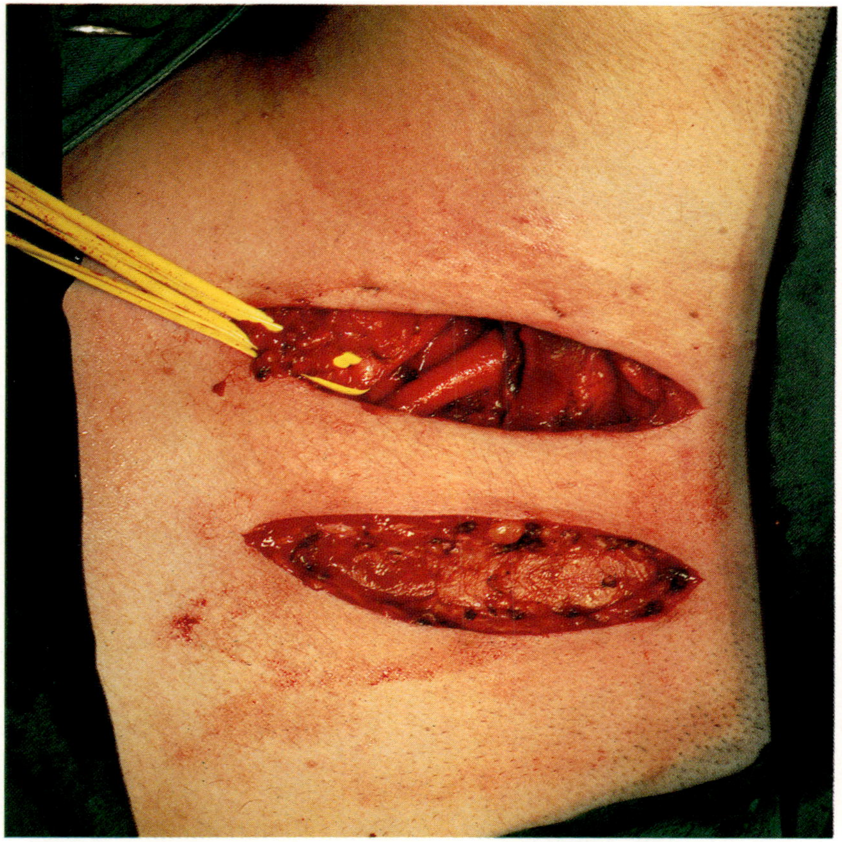

58

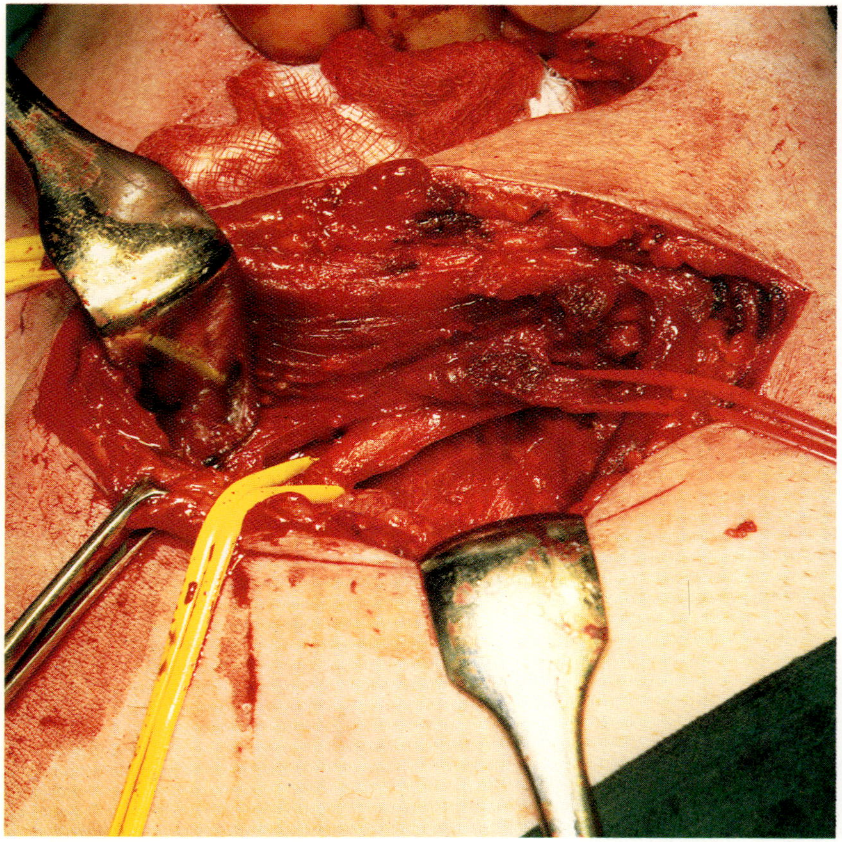

57 Infraclavicular stage of decompressing C8 and T1 roots, by excising the first rib. Infraclavicular incision from the sternum to the anterior border of the deltoid muscle.

58 The incision divides the deep fascia and cuts the clavicular fibres of the pectoralis major and the clavipectoral fascia. The subclavian vein is exposed lying on the medial horizontal part of the first rib. At the medial end of the dissection, the large tendon of the subclavius muscle is isolated with a sling and divided. **This step must be well exposed to avoid damaging the subclavian vein as it passes between the muscle and the first rib and in close proximity to the tendon.** The venous tributaries are ligated and divided to free the vein.

59

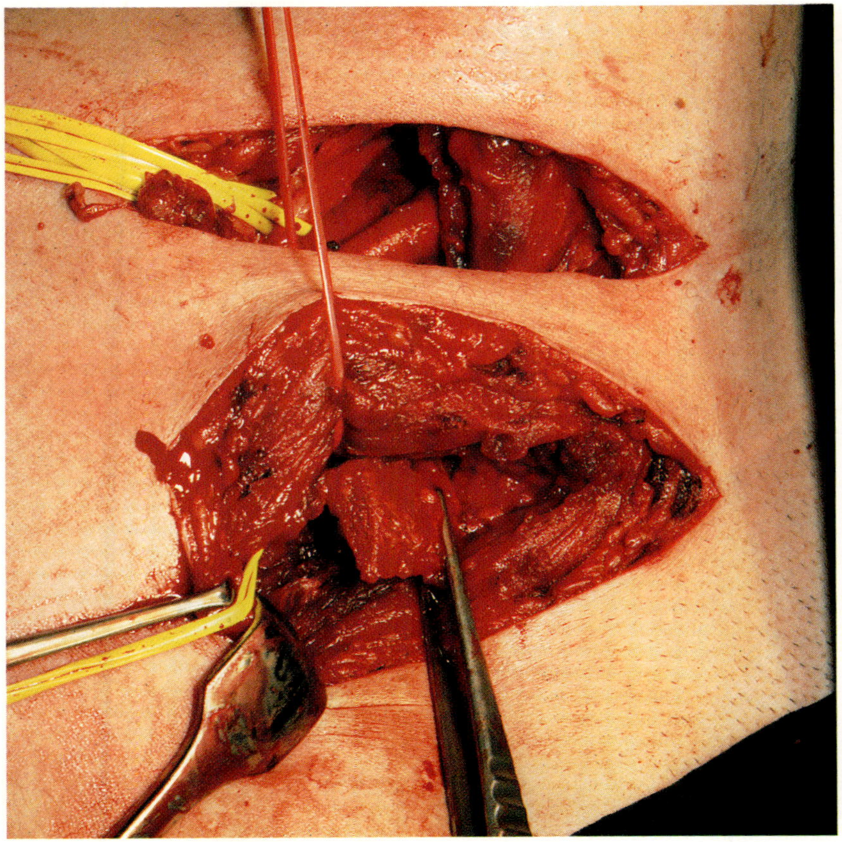

59 Protecting the third part of the axillary vein by lifting it off the first rib. The vein is lifted on a sling. The space behind the vein between the clavicle and the first rib is developed from above and below the clavicle. The intercostal muscles between the first and second ribs are cut and the lower border of the rib cleared.

The pleura is pushed away from the rib and retracted. This allows the first rib to be cut in the middle third with straight double-action bone cutters. The sternal attachment is cut and the anterior half of the rib removed.

60

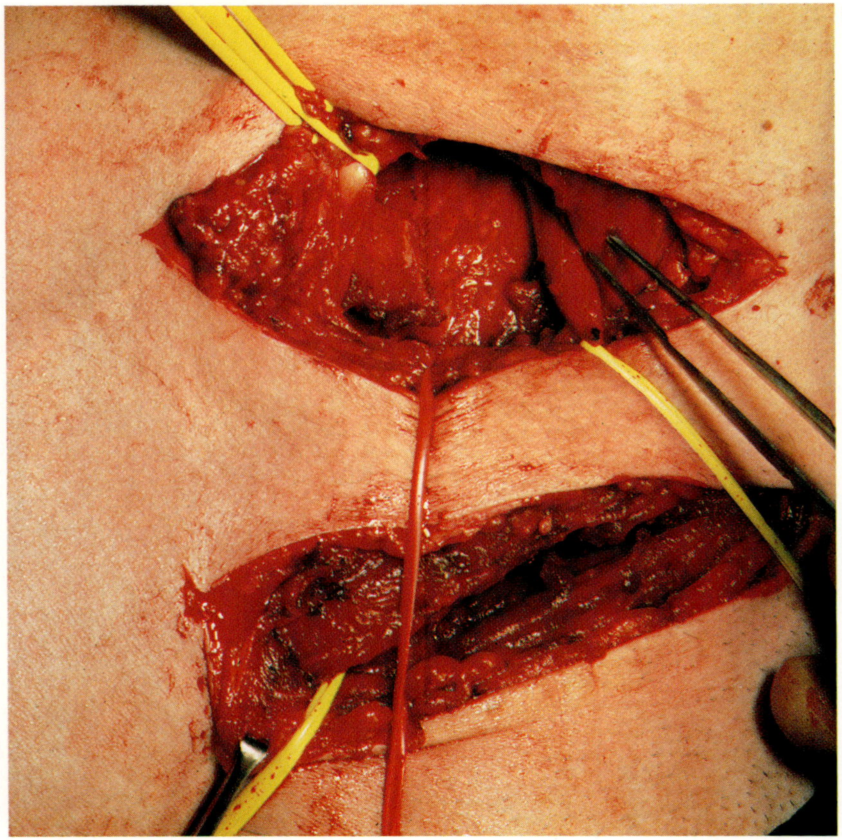

60 Posterior half of the rib above the clavicle. The posterior half of the rib is now free and seen clearly above the clavicle. Clearance of the lower border of the rib is continued from above. Traction on the anterior end helps this manoeuvre as the rib becomes more mobile.

A right-angled bone cutter is used to cut the rib at its neck, making sure the T1 root is posterior to the blades of the cutter.

61 Excision of posterior half of the first rib. The posterior half is removed easily. The neck of the rib is trimmed back beyond the T1 root with rongeurs.

61

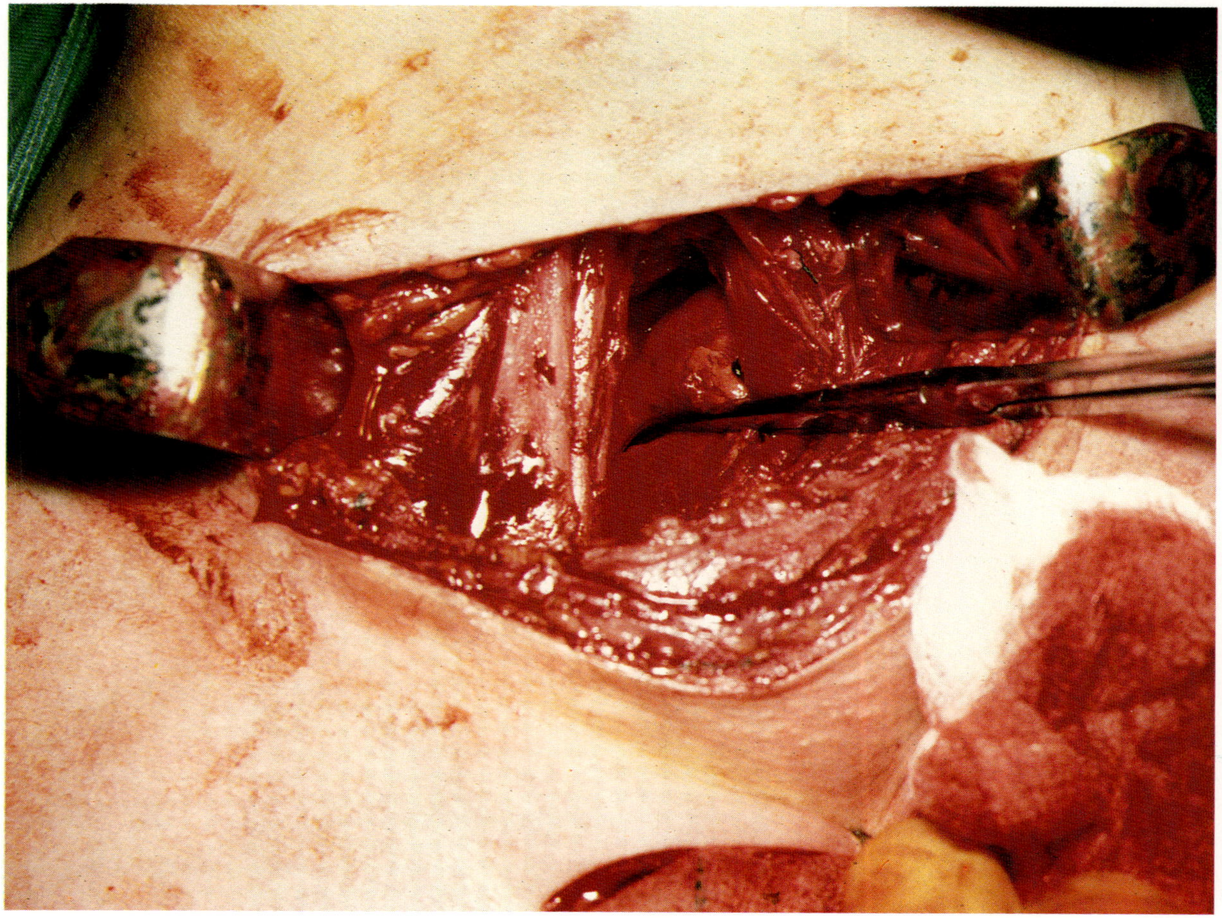

62

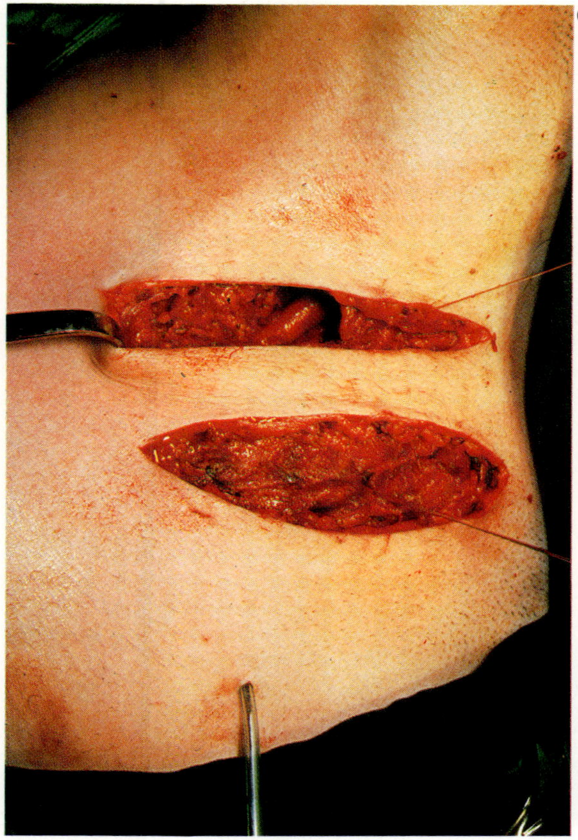

63

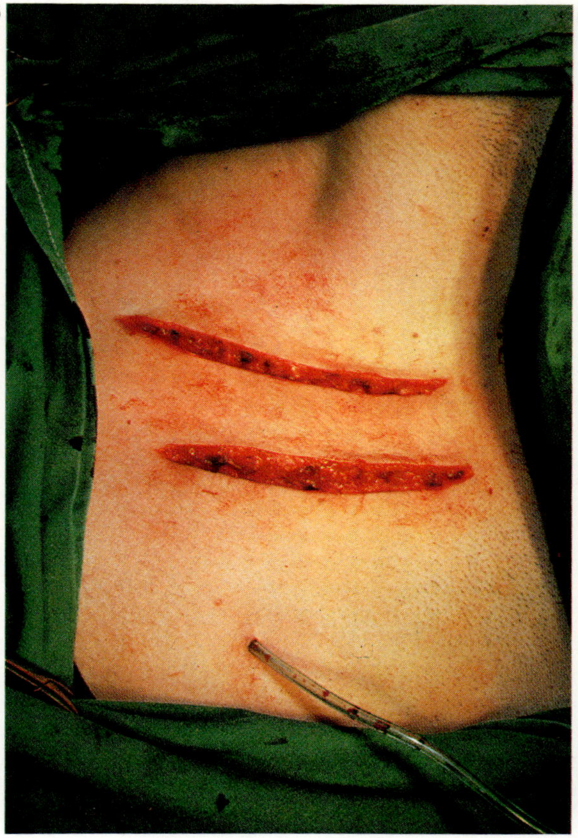

64

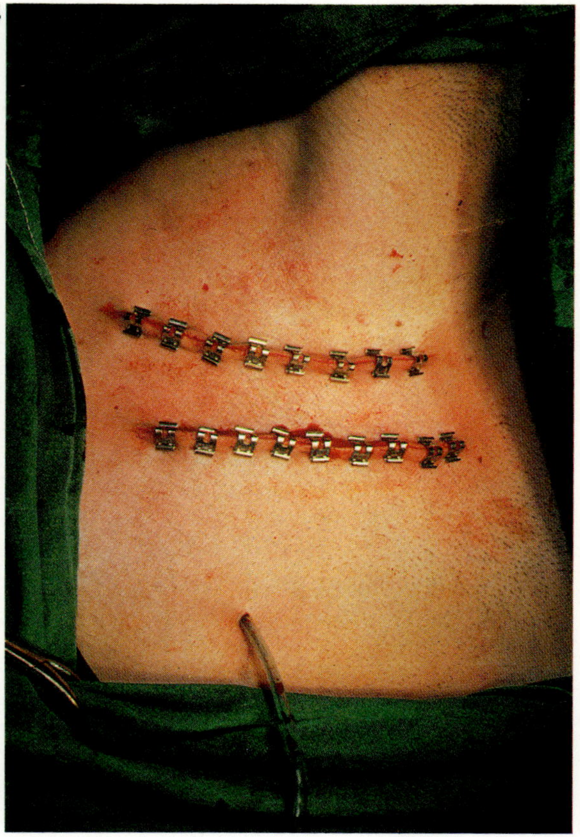

62 Drainage of the residual cavity. There will be oozing of blood from the cut muscles and a multipore drain is placed in the cavity emerging below the clavicle.

The clavicular head of the sternomastoid is resutured and the clavicular head of the pectoralis major is sutured using 1.0 chromic catgut.

63 Closure of the deeper layers. The platysma muscle above and the deep fascia below the clavicle are sutured with fine 3.0 plain catgut.

64 Closure of skin. The wound is closed with clips or subcuticular Dexon. The drain is removed in 24 hours, provided that the chest xray shows a well-expanded lung with no evidence of pneumothorax or an extrapleural haematoma. The arm is kept strapped to the side for three or four days and rested in a sling for four weeks.

Transaxillary resection of the first rib

Transaxillary resection of the first rib is one way of decompressing the thoracic outlet and was suggested by Claggett in 1962. It is a common operation in the USA and parts of Europe but rarely performed in the United Kingdom. However, it does have certain acceptable indications. The procedure was first described by Roos[5] and the steps have been clearly defined by him. He not only removes the first rib by this route but also tackles cervical ribs and carries out extrapleural cervicodorsal sympathectomy. The approach can be considered for cervicodorsal sympathectomy in hyperhidrosis as the resulting scar is almost invisible in the axilla.

The main indication for performing the operation in world literature, is for the relief of pain, mainly in the C8–T1 distribution. The selection of cases with pain only is not easy. All my cases are seen by an orthopaedic surgeon and a neurologist, as well as a vascular surgeon before a decision is made to remove the first rib.

The operation has a limited use in decompressing the subclavian artery in the absence of a cervical rib, and is only advised when one is convinced that the compression is entirely between the clavicle and the first rib.

Chronic intermitent compression of the subclavian vein between the clavicle, the subclavius muscle and the first rib is for me the main indication for this procedure and is successful in almost every case.

Dramatic relief of post-phlebitic symptoms have also been obtained after resection of the first rib.

65

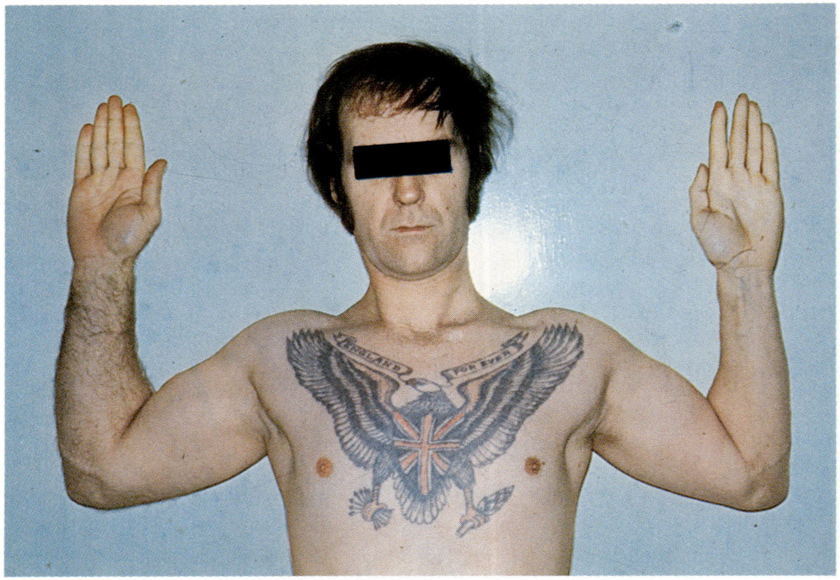

65 Pallor of the hand in arterial compression. Photograph of a patient in the Group 1 arterial compression showing pallor of the hand in abduction and external rotation to 90 degrees.

66

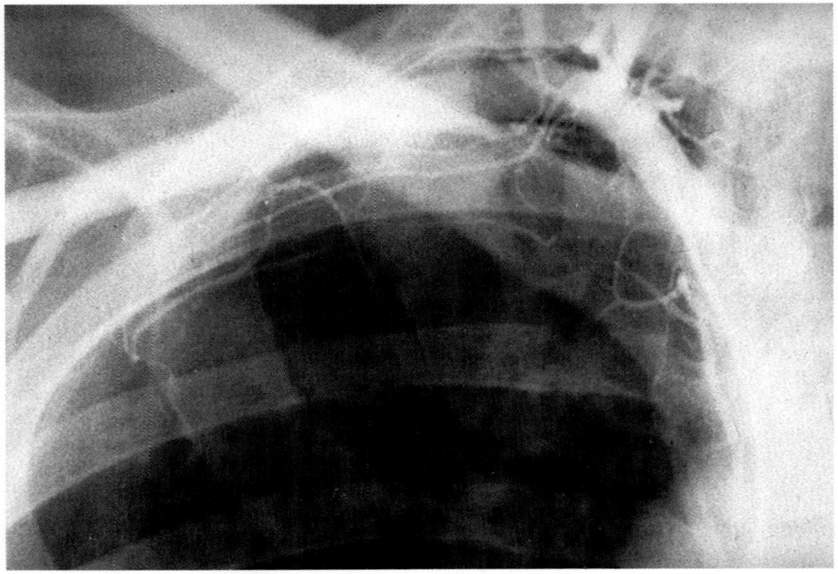

67

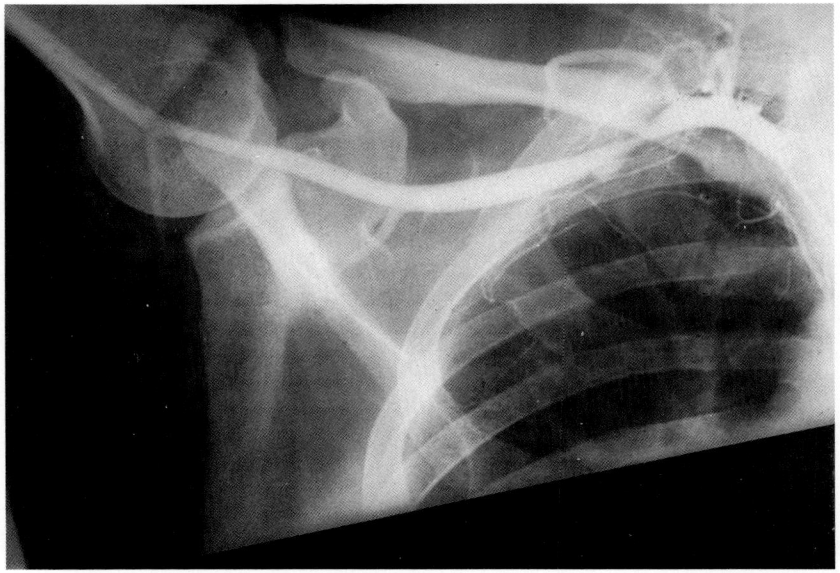

66 Aortogram in adduction. Arch aortogram showing the subclavian artery of normal calibre with the arm in adduction.

67 Aortogram in abduction. Arch aortogram demonstrating almost total occlusion of the subclavian artery with the arm in abduction.

68

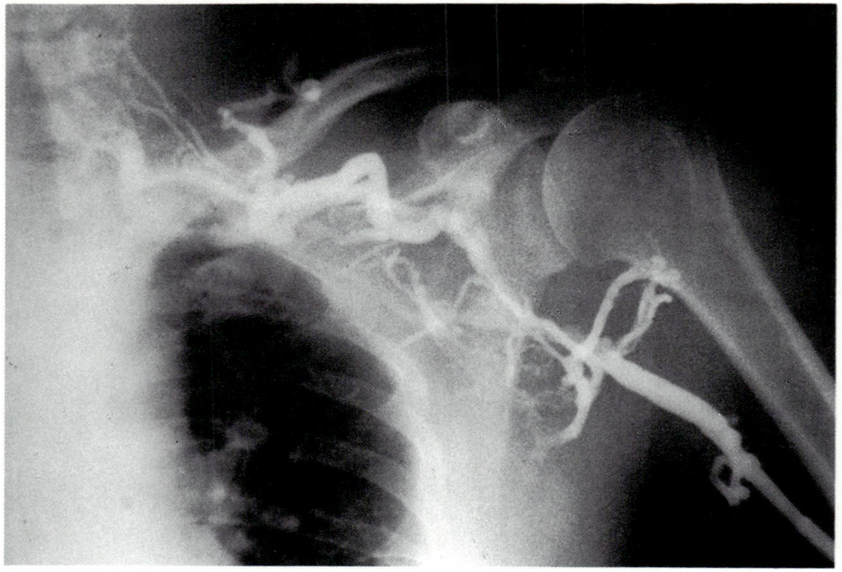

69

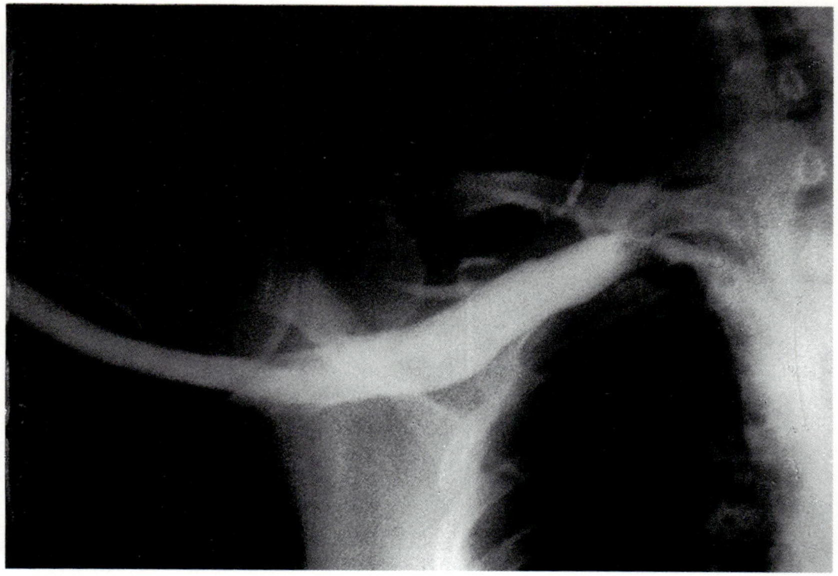

68 Post-phlebtic venogram. Brachial venogram showing post-phlebitic subclavian vein obstruction with collateral veins of varying sizes. The patient had functional disability of pain and oedema.

69 Venogram of opposite arm. Brachial venogram of the opposite side showing obstruction of the vein at the costoclavicular space with the arm in abduction. It is doubtful if thrombosis occurs in the absence of external compression.

70 Severe case of intermittent venous obstruction. Photograph of patient showing advanced stage of chronic intermittent venous obstruction with oedema and cyanosis of the hands. The symptoms are present in adduction as well as abduction.

70

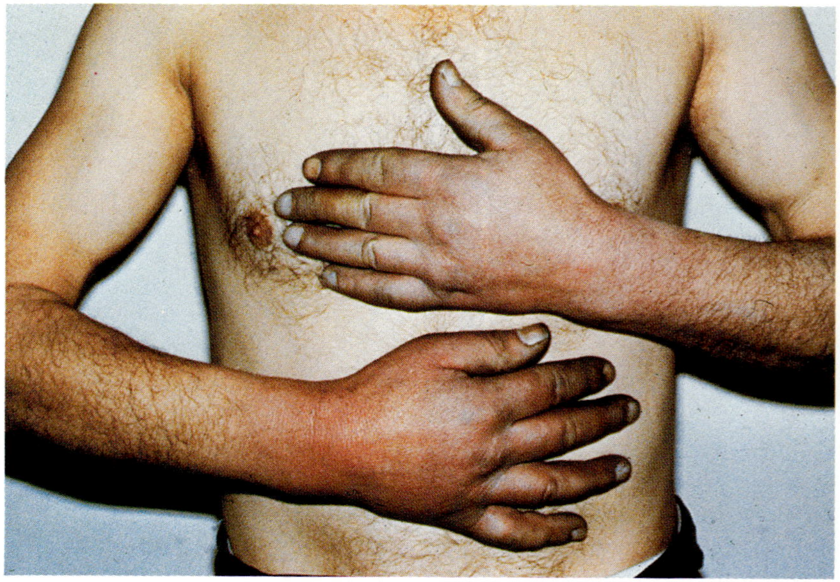

71

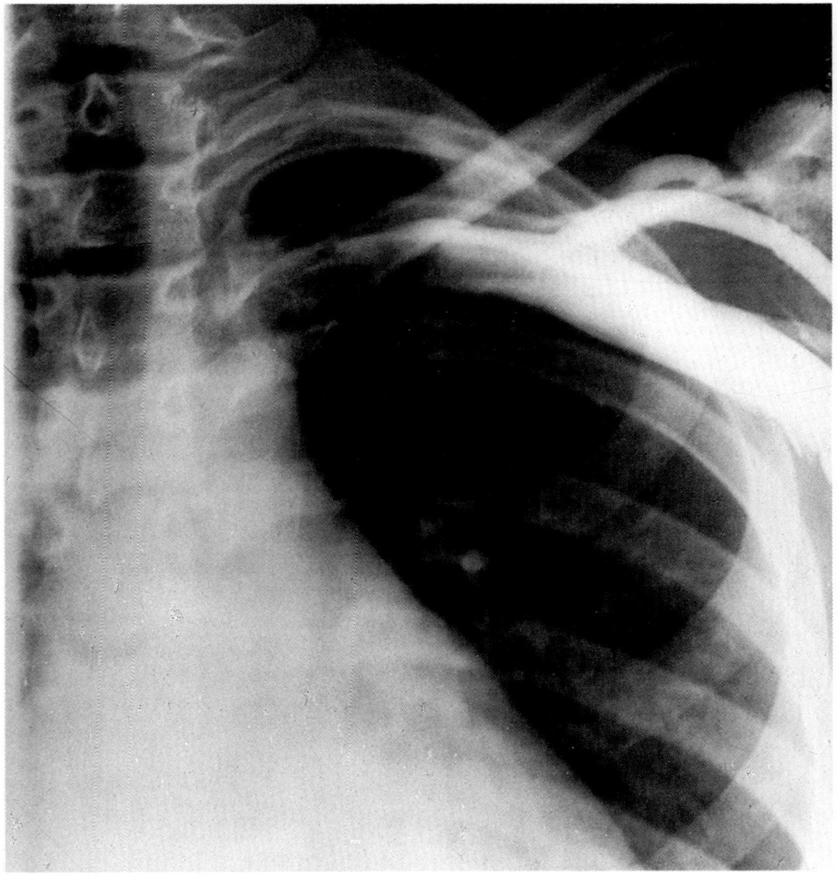

71 Venogram in chronic intermittent venous obstruction. Subclavian vein obstructed at the costoclavicular junction with the arm in adduction.

72

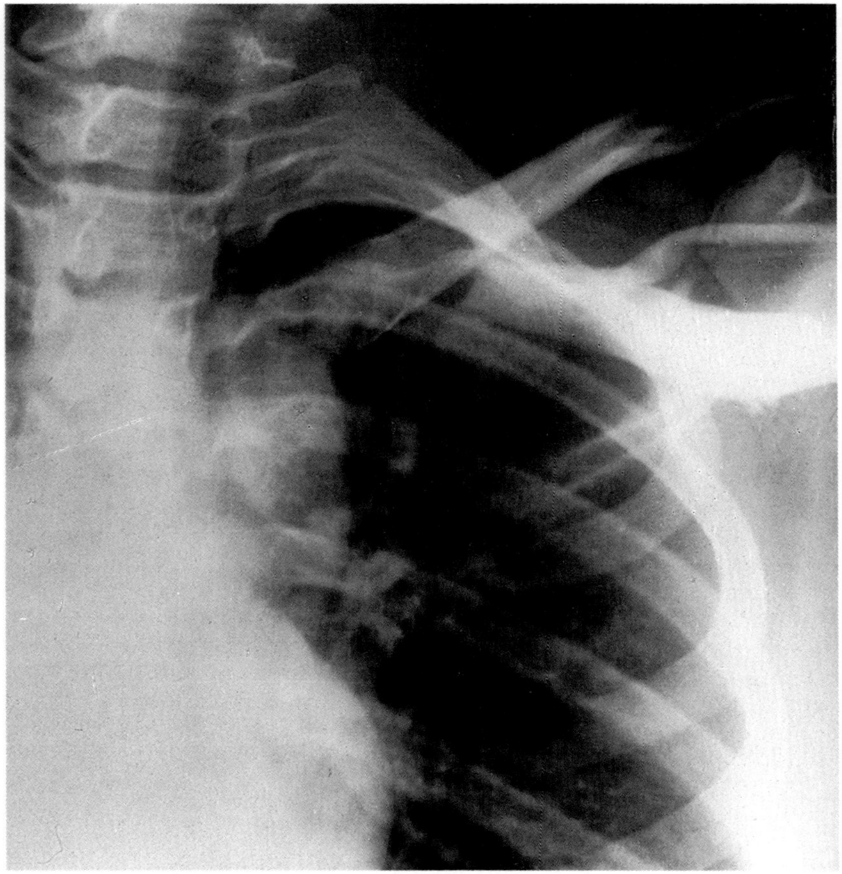

72 Subclavian vein obstructed with the arm in abduction.

73

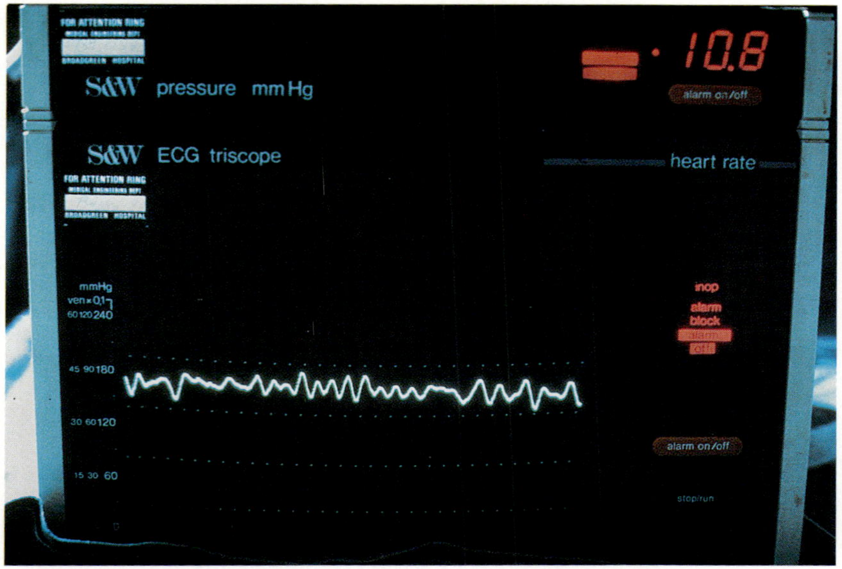

74

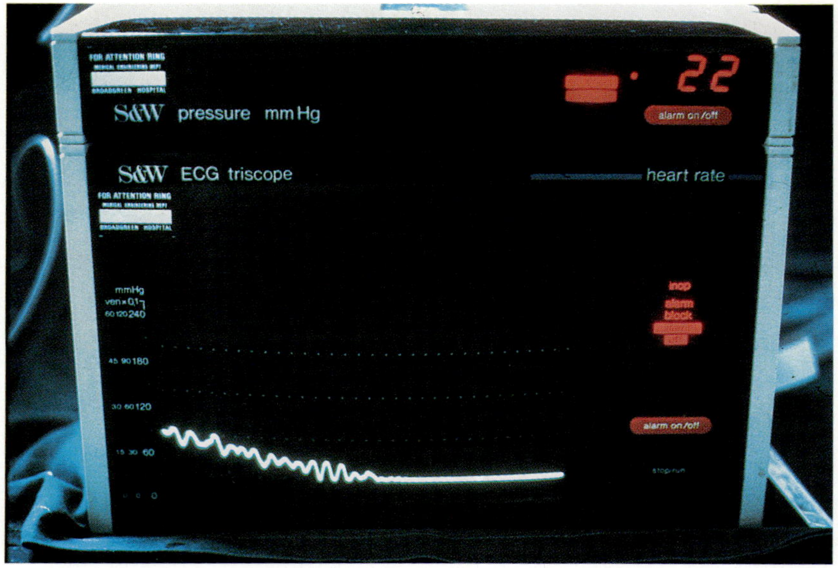

73 Venous flow and pressure recordings. Venous flow and pressure level with the arm in adduction.

74 Venous flow pattern shows complete obstruction when the arm is in abduction and during the same period the venous pressure is doubled.

75 Restoration of venous flow and lowering of venous pressure on returning the arm to the adducted position.

75

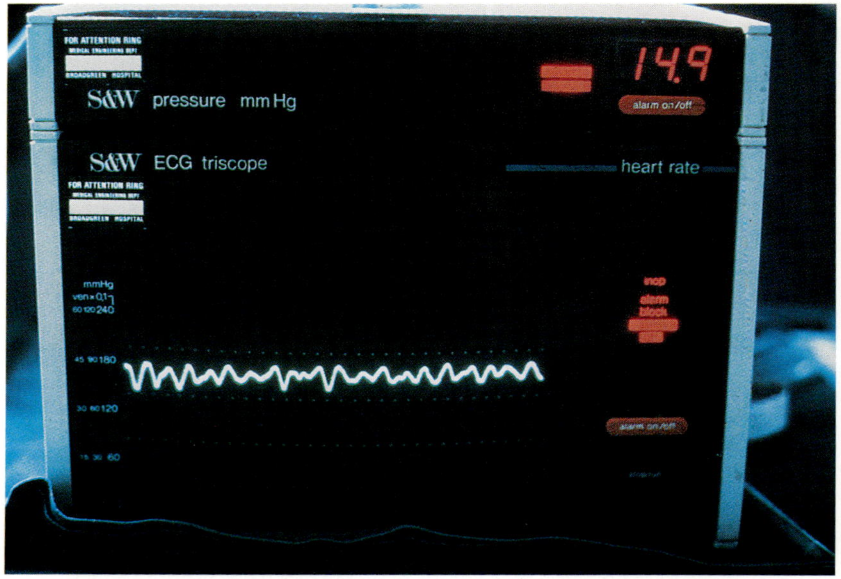

76

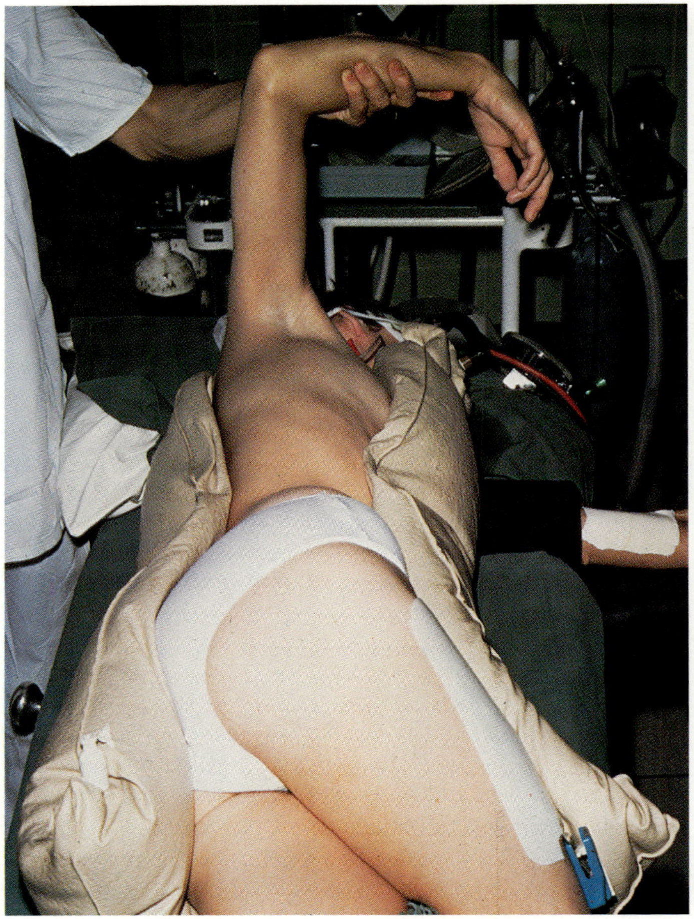

76 Position of the patient on the operating table. The patient is placed in the lateral position and conveniently supported by the Vac-pac surgical positioning system.

77

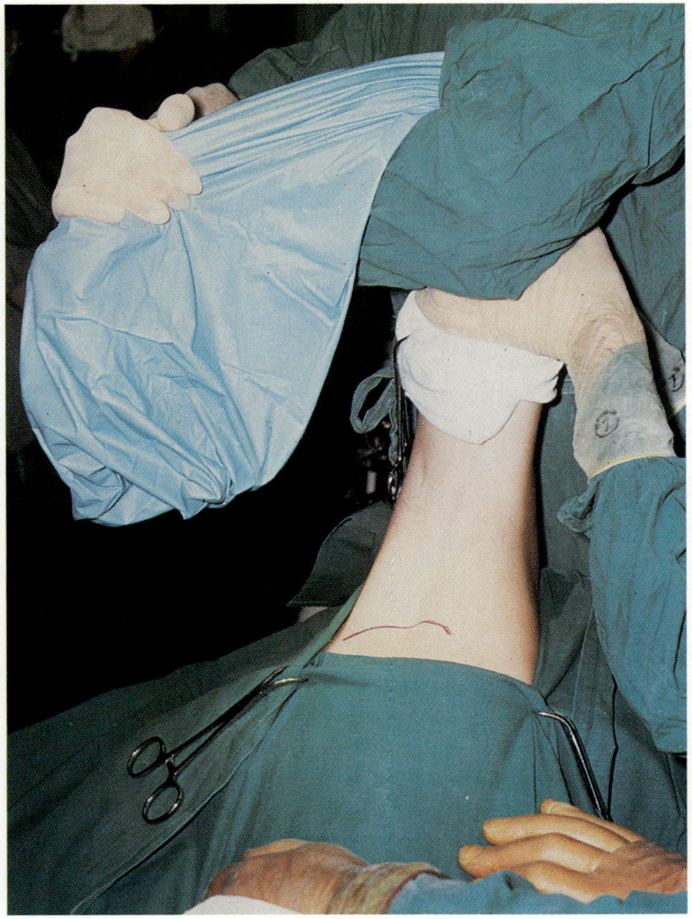

77 Arm-lock by assistant to exert leverage and open the axilla. An assistant holds the arm abducted 90 degrees at the shoulder, and flexed 90 degrees at the elbow, and leverage via an arm-lock can be applied to open out the axilla during surgery. The leverage is applied intermittently to avoid traction on the brachial plexus. Traction on the arm via a pulley can be used, but may be too forceful when dealing with women but quite useful when treating heavily muscled men.

78

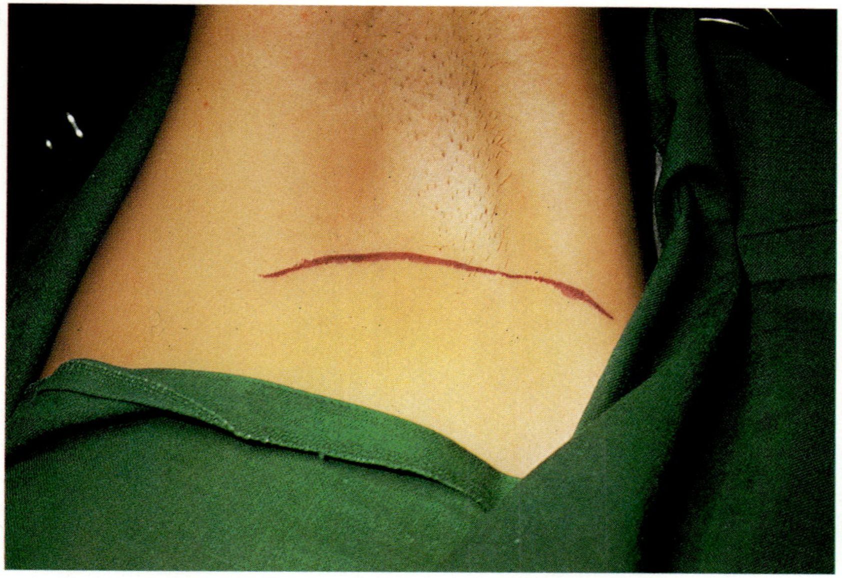

79

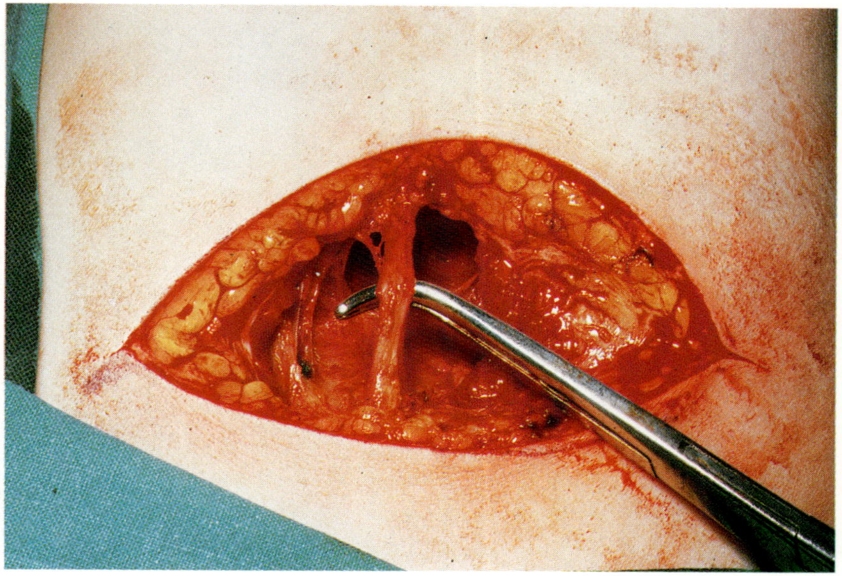

78 Incision. A curved 'smile' incision is made in the skin as it lifts from the chest-wall during traction. This usually corresponds to the level of the third rib.

79 Division of lateral thoracic artery and vein. The incision is deepened onto the chest-wall and the lateral thoracic artery and vein ligated and divided.

80 Opening out the axillary tunnel. A tunnel of loose connective tissue lies between the ribs and the axillary contents, and this is extended with blunt finger dissection. This plane can be missed if the incision is too high in the axilla and troublesome bleeding from axillary contents can occur.

80

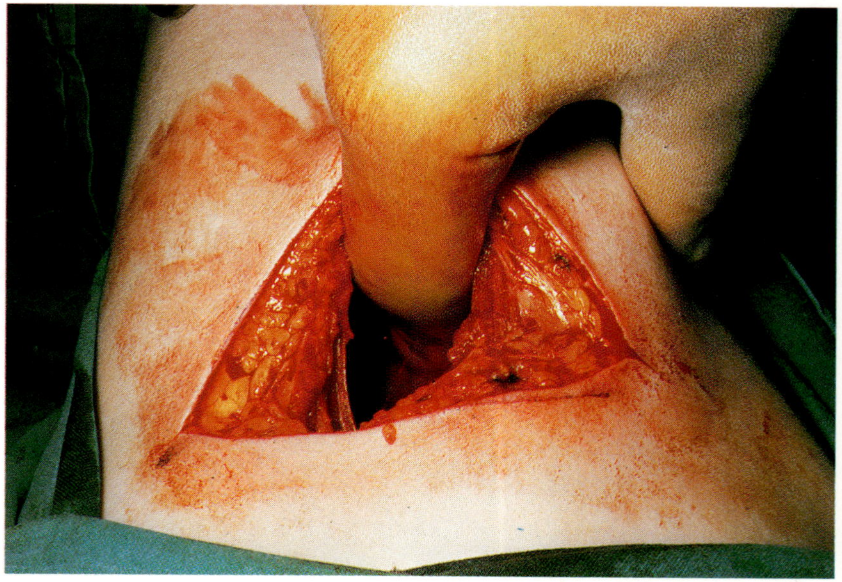

81

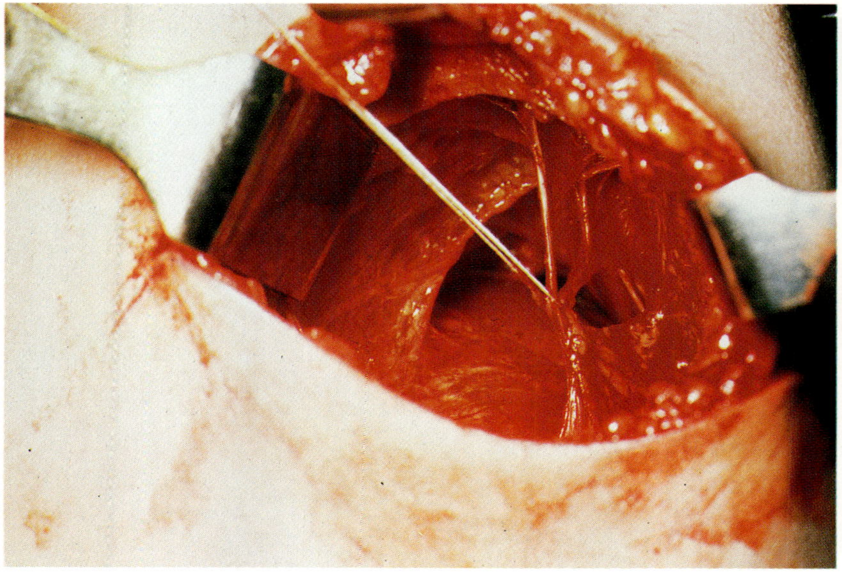

82

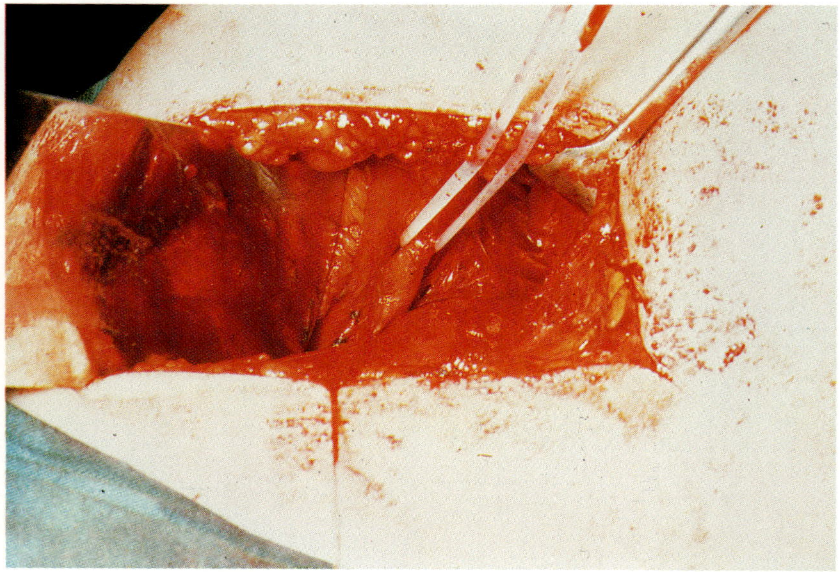

81 Protecting the intercostobrachial nerve. The intercostobrachial nerve passes from the second intercostal space to the medial aspect of the upper arm. The nerve is cleared with surrounding fat and connective tissue and retracted laterally. **Injury to the nerve leaves unpleasant numbness in the upper arm.**

82 View of the deep cavity showing vein, artery, and nerve. The first rib lies in the upper part of the tunnel; the subclavian artery, vein, and T1 nerve are seen passing directly upwards across the field.

83 Identification and division of the superior thoracic artery. A small artery – superior thoracic artery, a branch of the subclavian – must be identified, ligated and divided to avoid troublesome bleeding.

83

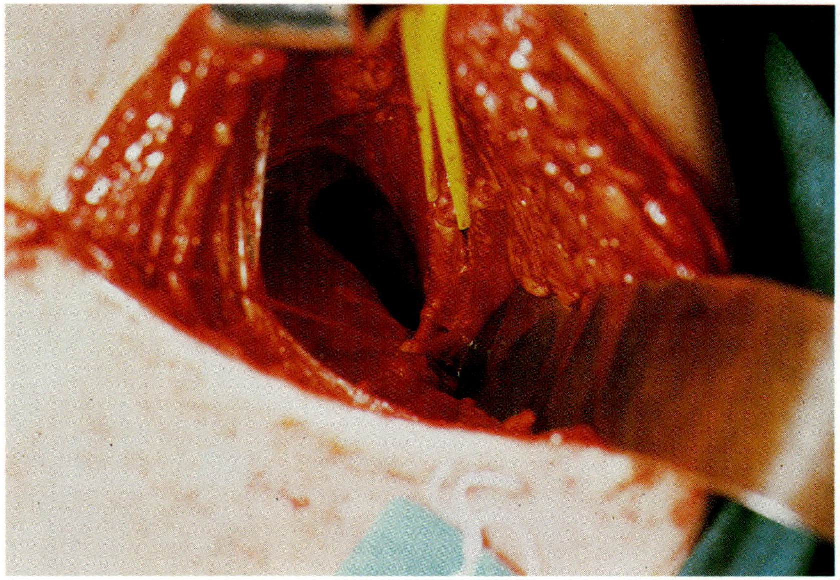

84

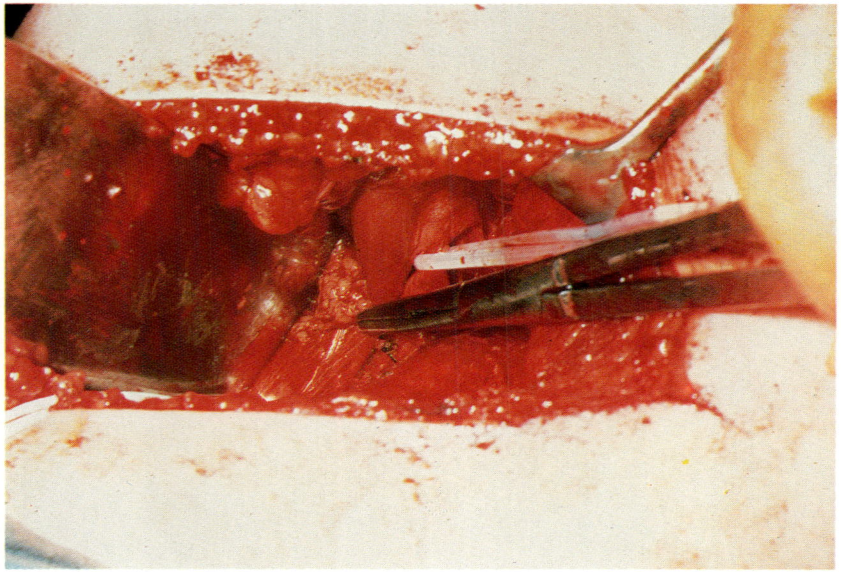

85

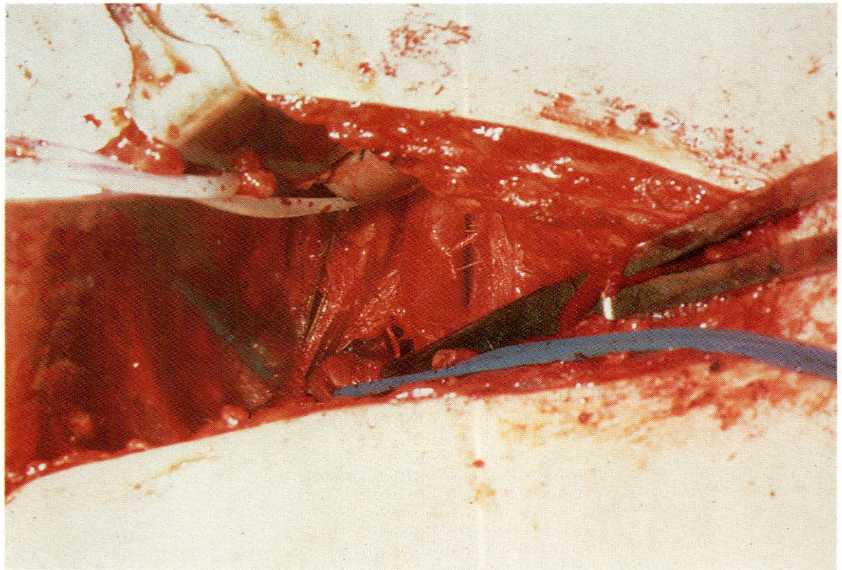

84 Exposure of the subclavius tendon in relation to the subclavian vein. The subclavian vein can be seen 'flapping' with inspiration and expiration. Immediately medial to the vein and parallel to it, is the thick yellow tendon of the subclavius muscle. This is dissected with utmost care and a space between it and the vein developed before dividing the tendon close to the rib.

85 Exposure of the scalenus anterior muscle attachment to the first rib. The vein and artery are freed gently from the upper border of the first rib. This helps the most difficult part in the procedure of the operation – the identification and division of the scalenus anterior muscle between the artery and vein. Blunt finger dissection between the artery and the muscle creates a space and a Lahey forceps can be hooked around the muscle. **It is divided near the rib to avoid injury to the phrenic nerve.**

86 Improved view of the vein, artery and nerve. After the scalenotomy Sibson's fascia is cleared from the upper border of the rib. The vein, artery and first thoracic nerve are now quite visible.

86

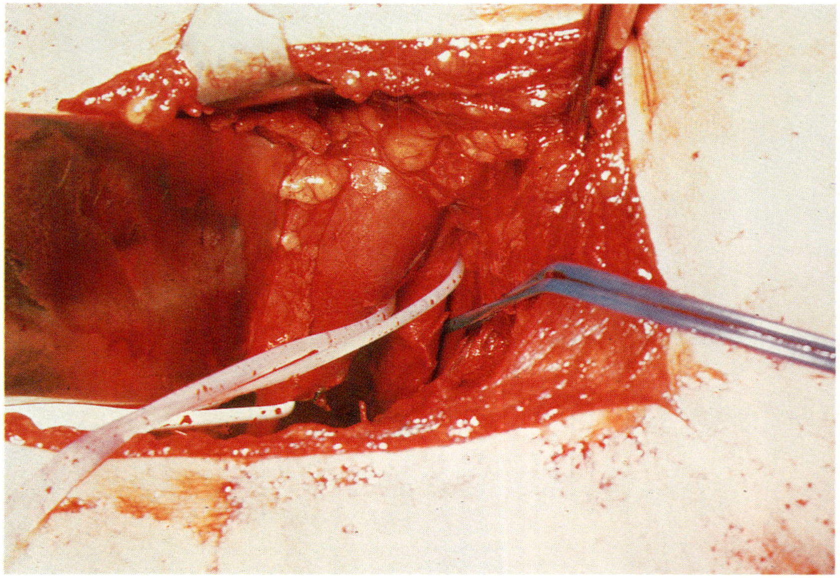

87

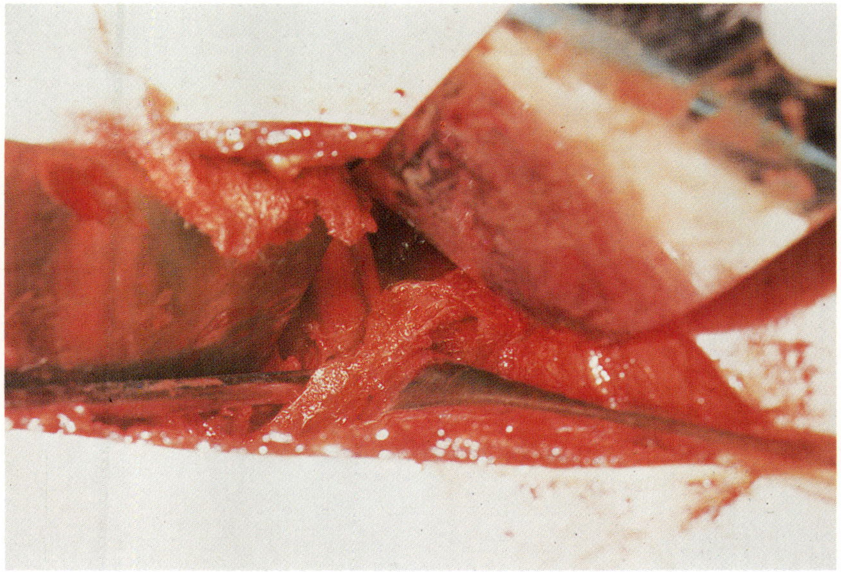

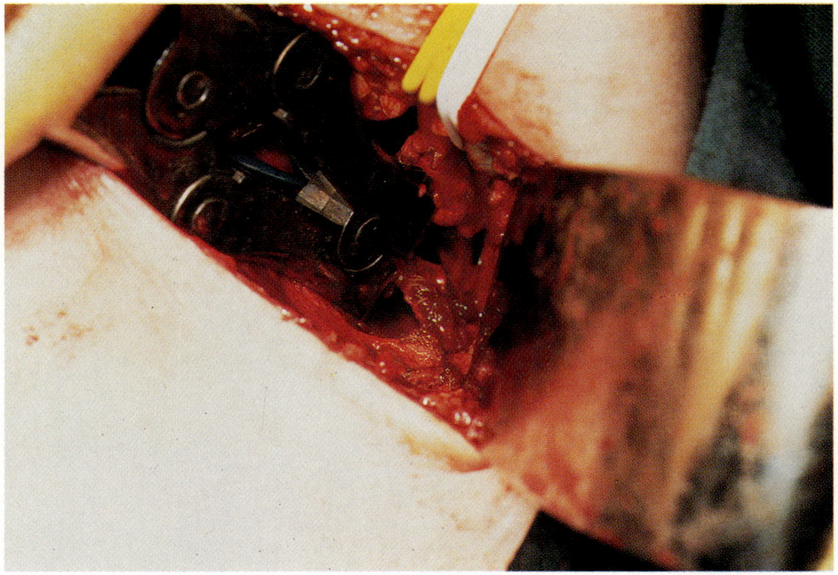

88

87 Freeing of the lower border of the first rib. The scalenus medius is stripped from the first rib posteriorly using a Morrison Davies rib raspatory or Overholt's raspatory; the intercostal muscles are divided and the stripper used to free the lower border of the rib from surrounding muscles. The pleura is pushed away gently from the rib and the finger can be passed behind the rib to finally clear the borders and make sure the whole rib is only attached at both ends.

88 Division of the first rib in the middle third. The rib can be removed in toto but a simpler method described by Urschel[6] is to divide the rib in the middle and as a first step remove the anterior half from its sternal attachment. The more difficult posterior half can now be managed more easily. The first thoracic nerve is dissected away from the neck of the rib and a narrow malleable copper retractor placed between the nerve and the rib. A right-angled double-action bone cutter is passed into the wound and the rib cut at its neck. Any remaining portion of the rib anterior to the first nerve is removed with rongeurs. Small spicules of bone must not be left to damage or irritate the nerve.

89

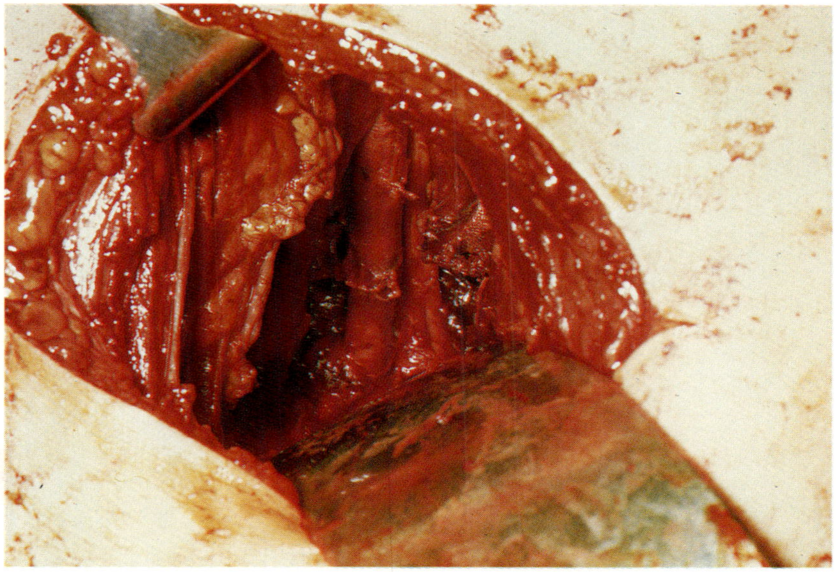

89 Post first rib resection view of the axilla. Wide exposure of the thoracic outlet after removal of the first rib. The vein, artery and nerve are viewed clearly as they traverse the space.

90

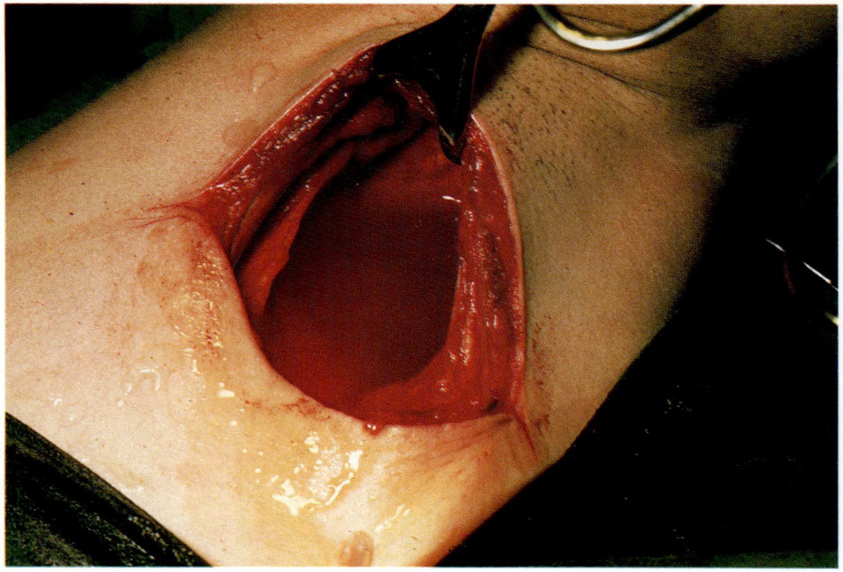

90 Post-excision check on haemostasis and pleura. Haemostasis is checked. The anaesthetist inflates the lung fully. **If there is no leak, the cavity is filled with saline to displace air which if left can be painful as surgical emphysema.** If there is pleural injury a ready-vac drain is placed in situ, and the saline omitted.

91

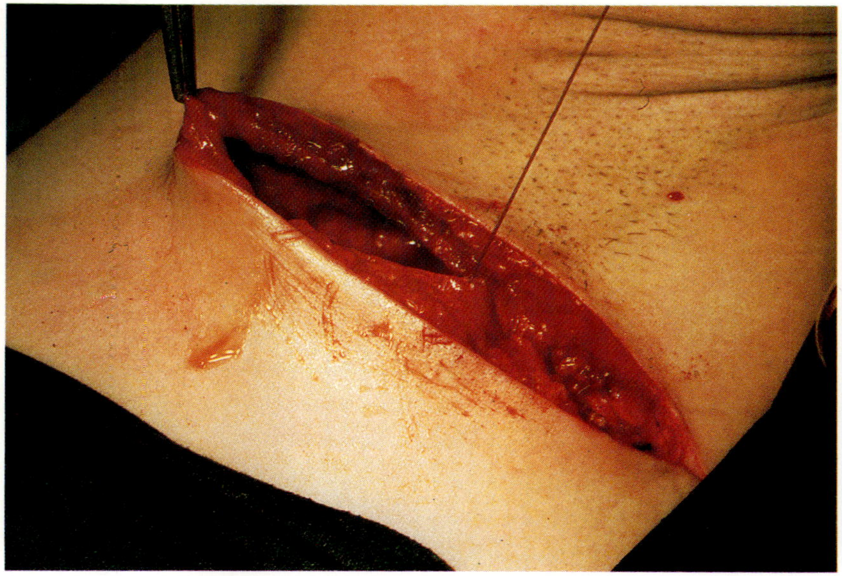

92

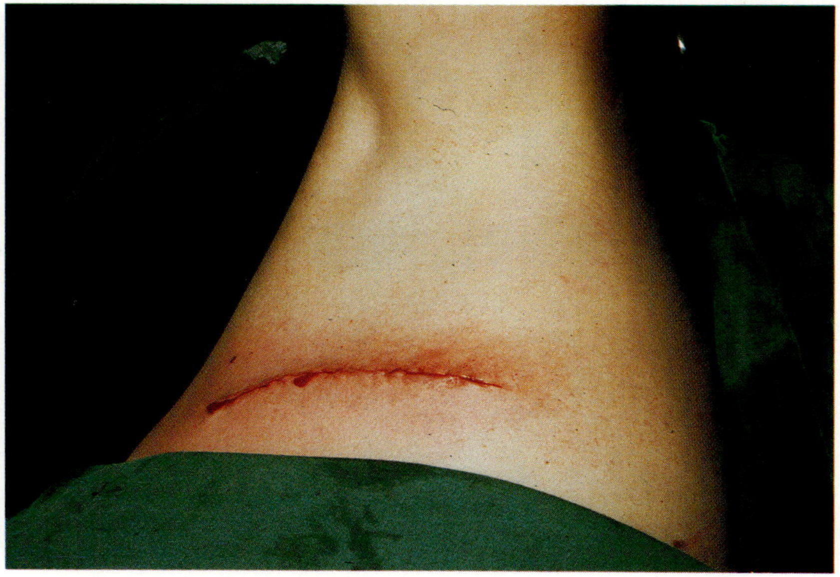

93

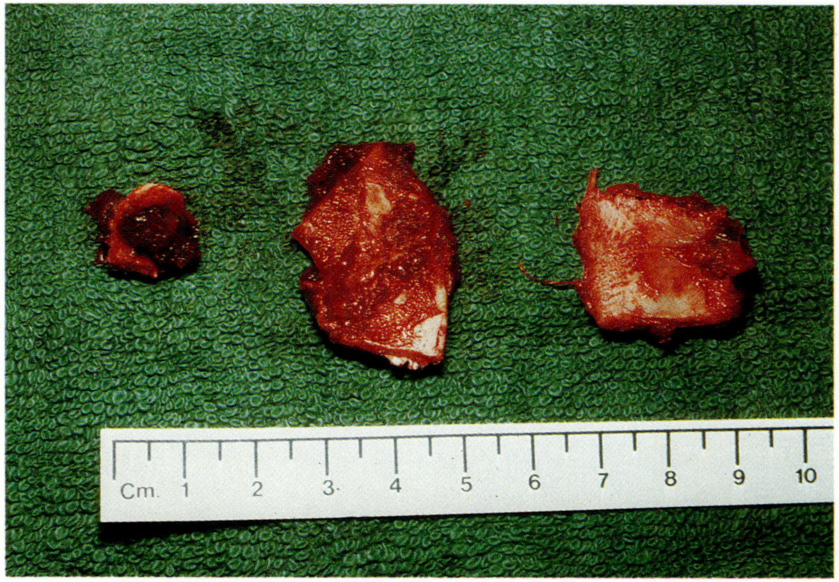

91 Closure. The subcutaneous tissues are sutured with continuous catgut.

92 The skin is sutured with subcuticular Dexon sutures or closed with clips.

93 Excised first rib. The first rib is excised in three parts – anterior half, posterior half, and the neck of the rib. The procedure adequately decompresses the thoracic outlet when there are no additional factors, such as cervical ribs or arterial lesions present. **When these demand surgery, the supraclavicular approach is safer for most general surgeons.**

References

1 Rob C.G. and Standeven A., 'Arterial occlusion complicating thoracic outlet compression syndrome.' *Brit. Med. J.*, (1958), **2**:709.

2 Clagett O.T., Presidential Address. Research and Prosearch. *J. Cardiovasc. Surg.*, (1962), **44**:153.

3 Stevenson I.M., Parry E.W., 'Radiological study of the aetiological factors in venous obstruction of the upper limb.' *J. Cardiovasc. Surg.*, (1975), **16**:580.

4 Short D.W., 'Cervical rib.' *J. Cardiovasc. Surg.*, (1975), **16**:135.

5 Roos D.B., 'Transaxillary approach for first rib resection to relieve thoracic outlet syndrome.' *Ann. Surg.*, (1966), **163**:354.

6 Urschel H.C., Razzuk, M.A., 'Current concepts. Management of the thoracic outlet syndrome.' *N. Eng. J. Med.*, (1972), **186**:1140.

Index

All figures are page numbers